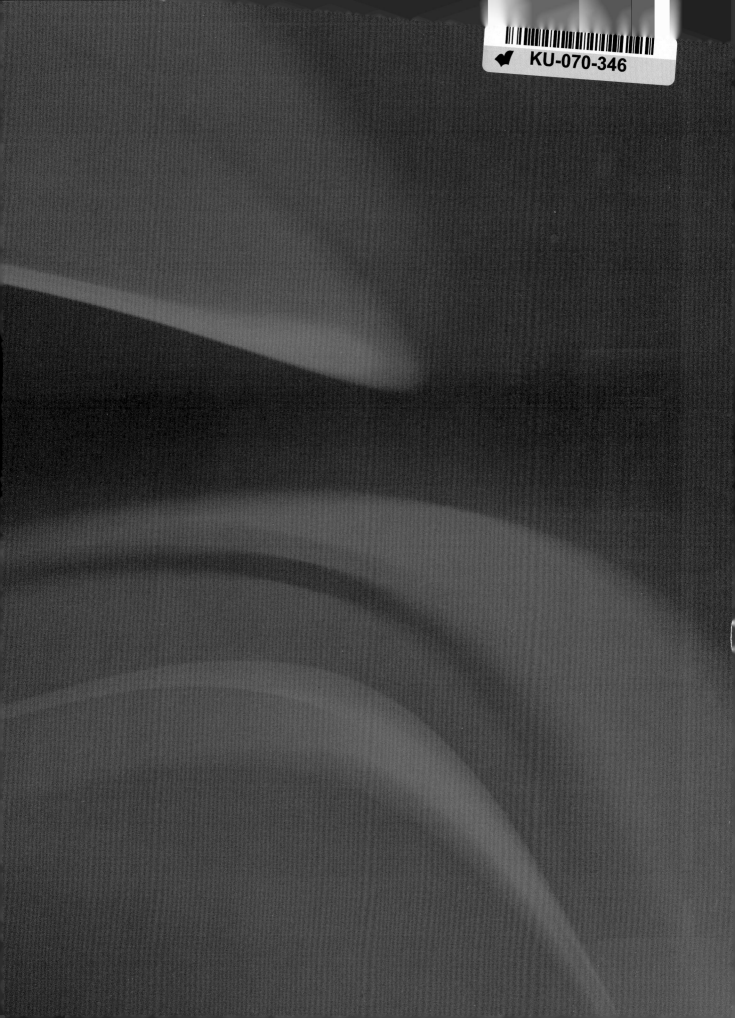
KU-070-346

Haynes

Body
Transformation
Manual

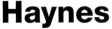

Haynes

Body
Transformation
Manual

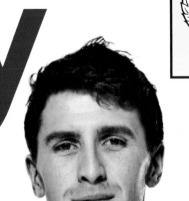

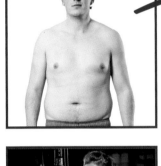

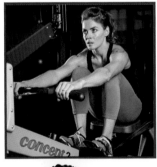

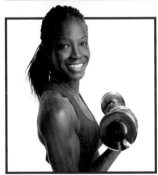

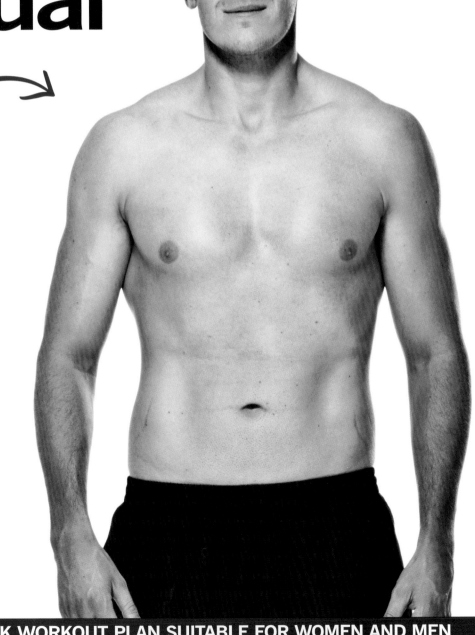

Sean Lerwill

THE ULTIMATE 12-WEEK WORKOUT PLAN SUITABLE FOR WOMEN AND MEN

© Sean Lerwill 2014

Sean Lerwill has asserted his right to be identified as the author of this work.

All rights reserved. No part of this publication may be reproduced or stored in a retrieval system or transmitted, in any form or by any means, electronic, mechanical, photocopying, recording or otherwise, without prior permission in writing from Haynes Publishing.

First published in December 2014

British Library Cataloguing in Publication Data
A catalogue record for this book is available from the British Library.

ISBN 978 0 85733 513 4

Library of Congress catalog card no. 2014942788

Published by Haynes Publishing,
Sparkford, Yeovil, Somerset BA22 7JJ, UK
Tel: 01963 442030 Fax: 01963 440001
Int. tel: +44 1963 442030 Int. fax: +44 1963 440001
E-mail: sales@haynes.co.uk
Website: www.haynes.co.uk

Haynes North America Inc.
861 Lawrence Drive, Newbury Park,
California 91320, USA

Printed and bound in the USA

While every effort is taken to ensure the accuracy of the information given in this book, no liability can be accepted by the author or publishers for any loss, damage or injury caused by errors in, or omissions from the information given.

Author:	Sean Lerwill
	(Twitter @seanlerwill)
Project manager:	Louise McIntyre
Copy editor:	Ian Heath
Design:	James Robertson
Photography:	Tom Miles
Stock photos:	Shutterstock

Contents

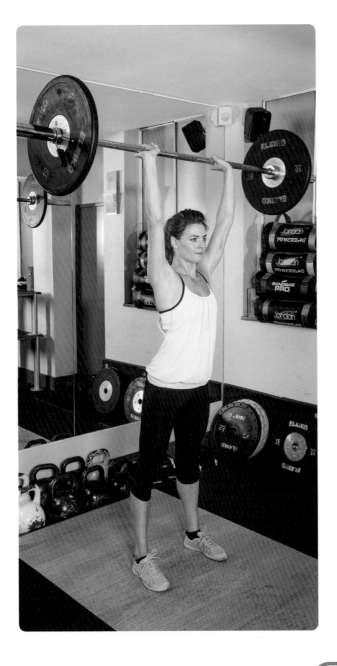

CHAPTER 1
INTRODUCTION

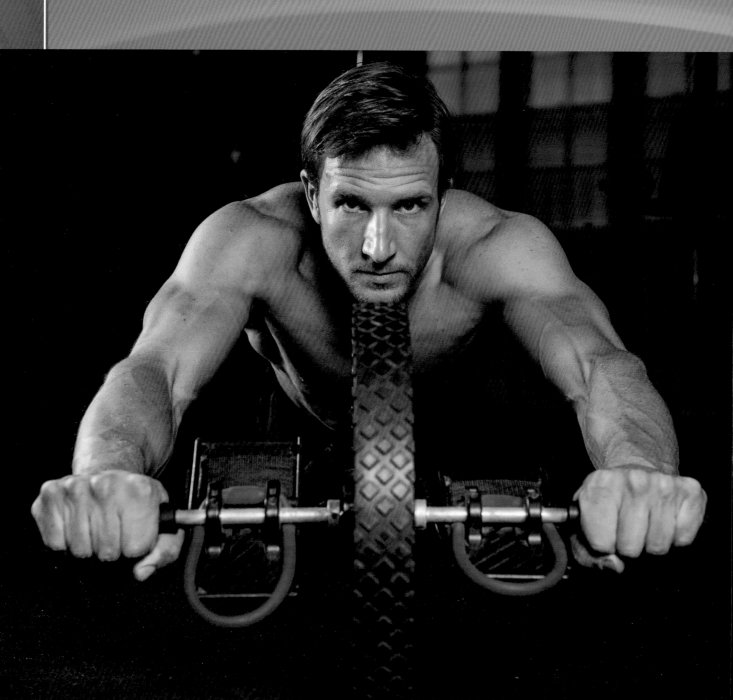

Welcome to the Haynes *Body Transformation Manual*. It contains pretty much everything you need to know and implement in order to achieve a body compositional change, by lowering body fat and increasing muscle to transform your physique or figure.

Metaphorically speaking...

As a teacher – in fact as a human being – I'm a big fan of metaphors. I think they're an invaluable tool for explaining things. Whether you're trying to get your point across to win an argument, or teaching a complete beginner in the gym, a metaphor can simply and quickly enable them to see (and often, more importantly, feel) your point of view, and understand what it is they're doing, not doing or trying to do.

When I found out this book had the go-ahead, I thought about the best way to introduce the subject. At first I thought about a meaningful paragraph on why we're obsessed with how we look; from Hollywood to *Heat* magazine, we have images of the 'perfect' figure or physique rammed down our throats almost daily, and we're all led to believe that *that's* how we should look. However, this seemed quite futile really, as if you're reading this you probably already know that. I'm not suggesting this is a bad thing at all – it's every individual's prerogative to want to look the best they can. Equally, if having an aesthetically pleasing figure or physique gives you confidence, inspires you and helps you become a fitter, happier human being, then personally I think that's great. I'm happy to admit that I'm close to addicted to exercise and training, eating healthily and keeping in good physical shape. It's not only a de-stresser for me, it earns me a living, as a writer, trainer, actor and cover model.

Anyway, back to my metaphor.

Attempting and completing a body compositional transformation is like writing a book. Firstly, it's most certainly a marathon, not a sprint. It's different for every single person, as their individual lives, experiences, lifestyles etc affect the process, and there's no set timescale for each person. It takes as long as it takes, although the more intensely you approach it and the more effort you put in, the more speedily you'll see results. Though not always *better* results. Writing a book and performing a transformation can both become all-encompassing, something

Have no fear of perfection – you'll never reach it

Salvador Dali

you think about at work, in bed and while trying to relax: they both become the focus of your life until they're complete. But – and this is the worrying thing for trainers and writers alike – you'll never be 100% happy with the results! You'll always feel something can be improved. And I guess it can.

I truly feel that this sums up what writing a book or undertaking a body transformation is all about.

So, I now have a question for you: are you willing to commit to this, 100%?

If you're thinking 'Well, maybe 80–90%,' then I'd advise you to put this book down until you can commit 100%. As a trainer, I've turned away clients who soon show that they can't commit. I train people online at distance, and often tell people to go away and sort their lives out before trying to do this. It's not something you can do half-heartedly, and I don't like wasting people's money or time, or come to that *my* time. Equally, every client I take on is a walking advert for me. Their failure reflects on me, and as an ex-Royal Marines Commando I don't like failure. Having said that, don't let fear of failure stop you from even starting; just be prepared to sort out your issues before starting in order to prevent failure from occurring.

Commit to this and I guarantee you'll look considerably different by the time you finish to how you look now. But you MUST commit 100%. If you have any delaying issues in your life, work, relationships etc, sort them out first, you don't need the stress ... in fact, we can't have you stressed: it could make you store body fat (yes, really! – read on to find out more).

Committed? Good, turn the page...

> **Don't be afraid to fail. Anything I've ever attempted, I was always willing to fail. You can't be paralysed by fear of failure or you will never push yourself. You keep pushing because you believe in yourself and in your vision and you know that it is the right thing to do, and success will come. So don't be afraid to fail.**

Arnold Schwarzenegger

What can you expect?

There are lots of training programmes, specials diets, fat burners etc out there for you to use, try, rave about or criticise. This book is trying to be different. I'm trying to 'KISS' – Keep It Simple, Stupid. I was a Royal Marine Commando, remember, and that's something we always tried to do. Why complicate things? Yes, there are a number of new and unique methods for changing people's physique, getting people fit, adding muscle, dropping fat and so on. However, the method laid out here is simple, and based around the basics of fitness and muscle building: progression, intensity, failure and variety. It therefore should maximise your body's ability to grow lean muscle and lose body fat – exactly what we want!

For that reason, although (hopefully) scientifically based (I have a BSc in Genetics), I'm not going to go into real depth over the reasons why we do things. I might give you a little insight, because, as someone who's a qualified teacher with a PGCE,

I believe education goes a long way to helping longevity of change; but I'm (hopefully again!) not going to bore you. I want this book to be like one of Haynes' car manuals: simple, easy to follow and, above all, useful.

In terms of changes, following the sort of programme and nutritional recommendations laid out it this book, men have gained up to 6kg of lean muscle with an average of 3kg, while losing body fat; around 6–9kg of fat can be lost (depending on how much you have to lose and how bad your starting point is, training and nutrition-wise).

Women can gain up to 4kg of muscle with an average of 2kg, while simultaneously losing around the same in fat, 4–5kg. This means you may weigh roughly the same, but as 1kg of fat takes up a larger mass than 1kg of muscle you'll be a tighter, firmer, aesthetically smaller person, despite weighing the same.

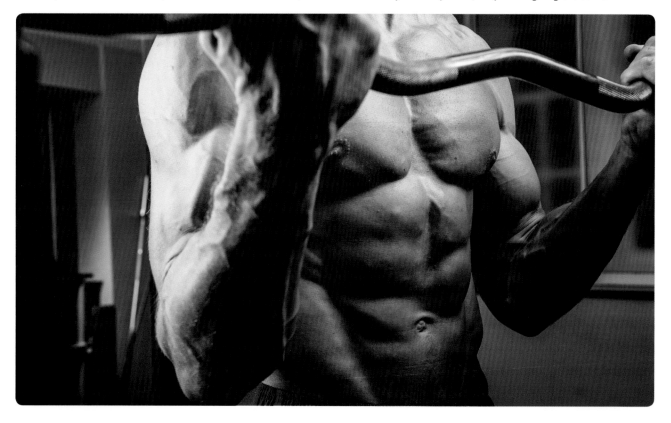

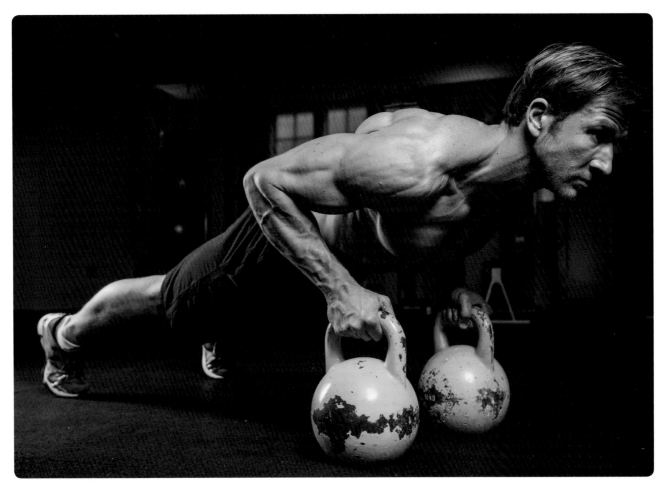

Training myths

Before we start, let's just get a few definitions sorted.

'Toning'

Many men, but even more women, state that they want to 'tone' or 'tone up'. Personally, I hate that word. It's misused in the world of fitness. Yet the industry is so wrapped up in it that I've been asked to comment on articles or write articles specifically mentioning how training will 'help tone' a woman. Unfortunately I must conform to get some good advice over, even if (to me) in a bad way.

However, this is my book, so I'm going to put the record straight. The word 'tone' is misused and misleading, yet it's so synonymous with what women want – or at least *think* they want – that it gets used all the time. As a scientific/medical term it can be best defined as follows: 'In physiology, medicine, and anatomy, muscle tone (residual muscle tension or *tonus*) is the continuous and passive partial contraction of the muscles, or the muscles' resistance to passive stretch during resting state.'

So we all already have muscles and muscle tone. If you didn't have muscles, you wouldn't be able to do anything physical. Walking down the stairs or nodding your head would be impossible. Therefore we all have muscle tone as well.

When someone says they want to tone up, what they actually want is to 'see' their muscles: see the definition/shape of those muscles. So if we all have muscle tone, why can't we see it? Simple. Because it's hiding under a nice layer of body fat. I'm not looking down on anyone here. I completely understand what you want. You simply believe your body isn't 'tight' or 'firm' and just want to 'tone it up' so that these 'wobbly bits' become 'nice and firm'. Well, that's body fat, and the only way to 'tone up' is to get rid of it. To do that you need to exercise and change the way you eat.

Turning water into wine and fat into muscle

Jesus supposedly turned water into wine. A miracle. Something that's impossible unless you're the son of God or a very skilled magician. Well, turning fat into muscle is the same. It's IMPOSSIBLE – and vice versa, while we're at it: you can't turn fat into muscle. You can't 'firm up' fat. It's fat. It's your portable comfort blanket and reminder that you eat more than you need and exercise less than you should.

Equally, if you build a little more muscle on this journey, then subsequently find it's hard to continue exercising to the same level, your muscle won't turn to fat either. There's no way it can happen. It's like me asking if your car will turn into a boat. Of course it won't. They're two different things. Always have been, always will be. You can get one, have both, lose one and lose both. But they can't become each other.

9

Happy so far?
A body compositional change will 'tone you up'

So, we now see that when people want to 'just tone up a little bit', they really want to see their muscles. It's actually the same as a man wanting to 'get ripped'. Both refer to a body composition change, a process of:

- Building new muscle while keeping existing muscle.
- Lowering body fat so that muscle can be seen.

On point 1, many people's training and way of eating means that they're breaking muscle down with too few calories and not enough protein, coupled with excess cardiovascular training. They're also slowing their metabolism by doing this. You'll see later that the exercise programme in this book has you doing far more resistance (weight) training. For men, this isn't a problem: they (usually) want to build some muscle. For women, though, the thought process is that weight training will make them too muscular. It won't.

Want to know a little secret? Victoria's Secret models do more weight training than cardiovascular training. They build muscle to ensure they have curvy, shapely legs that look good in the underwear they model. They do some cardiovascular training to keep fit and help lower body fat, but the large majority of their training involves weights, to sculpt their figures, build muscle and in turn burn body fat. Creating more muscle – which is metabolic tissue – also means they burn more calories day to day when not exercising.

Not convinced? Have you seen the pictures of overly skinny, almost skeletal people with absolutely no backside? They're that way because they've destroyed or broken down their muscle by cutting their calories way too low, performed no weight training and spent hours on end doing cardiovascular work. Their bodies, hearts and immune systems are in a bad way. It's not a good look and leaves them feeling drained, tired and looking gaunt and ill. I'm not chastising them, I feel sorry for them. I believe the High Street chain gyms should approach and help people who are obviously in this dangerous downward spiral. I don't want that for you. Hence I'm telling you now that muscle is your friend: it helps you move, work, play and stay alive longer. There are a whole host of health benefits linked to a healthy muscular body, like aiding you against osteoporosis and even some cancers. Ask any man what's more attractive: a female whose jeans have no backside to keep them up or a 'toned' bottom crafted in a gym squat rack? Forget it, you don't need to ask. You know the answer already.

Skinny girls look good in clothes, fit girls look good naked. I guess that's why Victoria's Secret models train with weights.

The final myth: targeting fat loss

You can't target fat loss. Simple. As much as we'd like to, we can't. You can do endless sit-ups or bench dips, but that'll never give you a six-pack or get rid of your bingo wings. So-called 'spot reduction' has been argued over for many years. Although some research now suggests that due to added blood flow to a specific area, spot reduction can aid fat loss, this only occurs once overall body fat is low enough. Therefore in general it's still regarded as a physiological impossibility.

The human body metabolises fat from the easiest places first, leaving the areas we consider 'stubborn' (such as the lower abdominal region) until last. So, if you're someone who's really concerned with getting thinner thighs or a flat stomach, you have to realise that this 'stubborn' fat probably won't shift until your overall body fat is low enough that the body is forced to utilise it. This would be around 10–14% in men and 15–18% in females. So, you can't just simply hit the gym and exercise the areas you want to look better, you have to see the bigger picture: exercise the whole body, feed it well and see the big changes overall as well as the little changes in the areas you dislike.

Simply put, you need to train hard and supply your body with everything it needs (nutrition, sleep, rest) while maintaining a calorific deficit. Then the body fat will be used as fuel and hence come off. But your body will still choose where it comes from and in what order, and your individual hormones and genetics play a huge part in this. As hard as you train, as good as your diet may be and whatever 'magic' fat-burning pills you take, you can't change that.

'I don't want to get big!'

Guys generally don't have a problem with getting bigger muscles, so this bit is for girls (and those guys that *do* have a phobia of growing). Don't fear using heavier weights. You won't grow 'too much'. For one thing, it's tough to grow – especially for girls. Those that do bodybuild train really, really hard, and most take substances to help them grow. Furthermore, if I'd created a programme and nutritional plan that could exceed the upper limit of 4kg muscle gain for women, 6kg for men, over 12 weeks (with the equivalent fat loss) I'd be a millionaire. Sadly, I'm not.

Still not convinced? Girls, how heavy is your handbag? The one you lug to work or the shops every day. About 10kg? Weigh it. You lug that around for hours on end, not just for one hour in the gym, yet you don't have one big arm or shoulder. You may have backache, though. (While we're on this, get a rucksack, not a large handbag. You'll thank me when you're 50.)

See what I'm saying? You'll be exercising your whole body, not just one arm with a handbag; you won't get big. You'll strengthen all your muscles, burn loads of calories and burn body fat. Having said that, it's a slow process. It happens over weeks, not days. Think of obtaining your 'toned' body as marathon training, not an overnight sprint.

Moving on

I'm hoping that by now you're intrigued, slightly better educated, and excited and ready to get under way. If you aren't, I apologise. If you are, perfect. Either way, turn the page. Let's get your body transformation started.

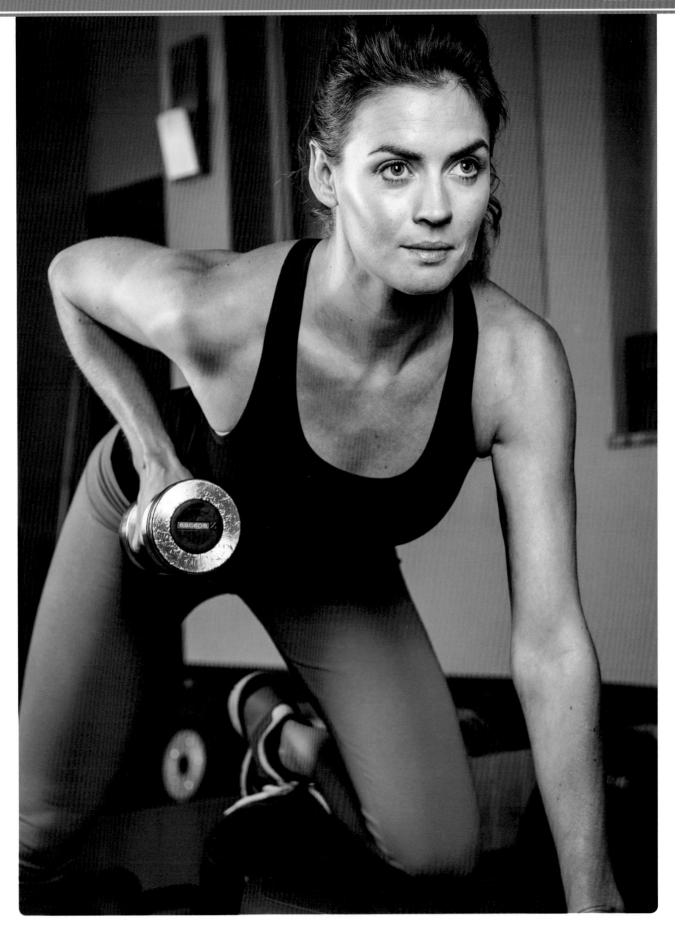

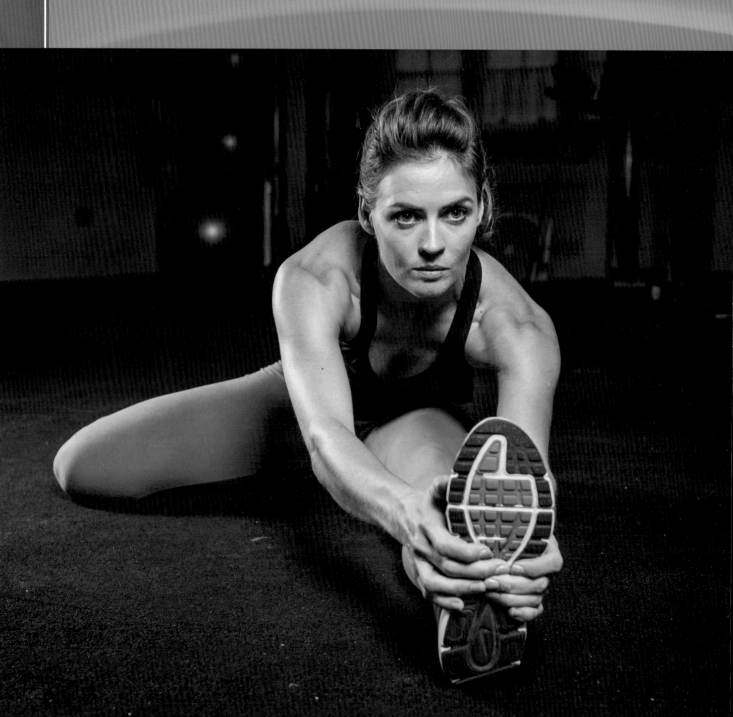

CHAPTER 2
STARTING OUT

The hardest part with a lot of things is getting started. Think about it. Anything you've ever dreaded: the first day at school, opening your credit card bill, breaking up with someone. It's the thought of doing it that's worst. It keeps you awake at night, gives you those butterflies in your abdominal area (yes, you have abs, they're just hidden – at the moment).

Once you face the thing that you have to do, it's hardly ever as bad as you expected. It's the same for making a healthy change and embarking on a body transformation. The thought of what's to come is far worse than the reality.

Going hand in hand with the above is the first training session, and, let's be honest, it'll be hard. Not as hard as you think it'll be (probably), but tough nonetheless. The thing is, once it's done then in a sense the worst is over. Your body will now start to change, to adapt, as will your brain and mental strength. I often say 'the first session is the worst': it's full of angst, expectation and worry, but once it's complete you kind of know what to expect, and from then on in you get fitter as the sessions get harder. Your mental strength and ability to push yourself get better as the sessions get tougher, so strangely things seem to get easier.

Tools for your toolbox

Throughout this book I'll try to impart a few gems of knowledge, or 'tools' for your toolbox, that I've gathered and believe are invaluable for you to get what you want from this process. That said, the set of tools is actually different for everyone. Yes, a few are needed by almost everybody, and we'll come on to those, but there are many that are individual-specific. Some people will already have them, but for others it'll be a case of reading everything laid out before them and following the overall plan while at the same time giving consideration to why you're doing what you're doing and what it is that you specifically need to do to achieve the changes you desire.

A tool for all: willpower

Simple. No arguments. Call it motivation, call it strength of mind (as the most recent Royal Marines Commando advertising campaign did), call it what you will, but you get the point. Without it, this won't work. I repeat, without willpower, this *won't* work, whether it's the willpower to get up before work and do a run, or the willpower to go out with a group of friends and not drink alcohol (yes, it is possible, and a genuine option).

At the end of the day, you've bought my book. I've written it, so my hard work is done. I have a physique and healthy lifestyle that I'm happy with. I'm content with having done my part, so it's no longer my job to force you to do anything. I'm happy. If YOU want this, if YOU want to make a change, only you can. Yes, you can train with a partner or friend. Yes, you can employ a personal trainer (though many are pretty poor at what they do). But at the end of the day it's down to you. If you want something, YOU have to go get it.

So, do you want it? It's not going to be easy. If you don't think you're ready, then stop now. If you aren't prepared to cut the desserts out, stop drinking and make time to train, then don't read any further. If you are, then read on.

I'm going to speak now about one tool that I've used with clients who do some of their training with me and some on their own. Separately, they've told me how when they feel like quitting early, or giving up, or not going to the gym, somehow they hear my voice (just as they would in a session) encouraging and helping them complete what's necessary. I've coined this their 'LerWill'. Yes, it's stupid and corny, maybe even slightly

You can't trust other people. If it's important, you have to do it yourself.

Neil Gaiman

Achievement is talent plus preparation.

Malcolm Gladwell

egotistical, but I've found it works. If I pop into your head every time you doubt yourself, every time you feel like giving up or staying in bed or having a chocolate bar, then who cares: it works, and it works because though it's kind of stupid, it sticks in their minds, and people remember it.

I want you to develop the sort of willpower that every Commando I worked with in my career, and every Commando that's ever existed has had. A true strength of mind to get on with it and work hard for what you want. A work ethic unrivalled by anyone else in your gym. The reason every Marine has that willpower is, I believe, twofold:

- They want their green beret so badly that they learn anything's worth putting up with.
- They don't want to let themselves, their brothers-in-arms or their teachers down.

Employ the same approach. *Want* this body transformation, and tell people you're doing it so that you won't let them down. Or me.

Goal setting: smart training

The acronym SMART is a good way of putting your goals into effect. It ensures they're not only thought out and fully considered, but are realistic and achievable as well. Hence SMART stands for:

S – Specific
M – Measurable
A – Achievable
R – Realistic
T – Timed

Specific

'Specific' means that your goal must be specific and not general. What I mean by this is not just saying 'I want to get fit.' That's not specific enough, so you'll lose track or get halfway to your goal and think 'That'll do'. 'That'll do' will NEVER do – remember that, and apply it in your everyday life every day.

The key is to be specific. How fit do you want to be? Fit for what? What you want is to improve your physique or figure. That gives you a real, specific goal, a tangible bull's-eye to aim for, one that, with hard work and dedication you WILL reach, and will be proud of yourself for doing so.

Measurable

This goes hand in hand with specific: by knowing you want a body transformation that allows you to fit into a specific dress or waist size, your goal becomes measurable. For example, saying your goal is 'to be fitter by a certain date' isn't measurable, whereas saying you want to be able to do ten pull-ups by 1 July is. So set your measurable goals, aim for them, and if you don't quite make them, oh well, no one ever learnt anything by getting everything they wanted first time. Even if you don't quite make your goal by the parameters you set, believe me, you'll have made far more progress than if you didn't set any parameters in the first place.

Achievable

Simple really: when setting a goal it must be achievable. For example, if (as in a real email I received) you're a man currently weighing 60kg, there's no way you can reach 90kg for the rugby season in three months' time. I'd be kidding myself if I told you that you could. That person may well be able to reach 90kg one day (depending on their height, genetics and of course drive, ambition and work ethic), but it's not achievable in three months. Equally, there are certain things that are unachievable for some people. Be sensible, be honest with yourself, but equally don't set the bar too low. There's a big difference between making life easy for yourself and setting achievable goals.

Realistic

Realistic goals go hand in hand with achievable goals. Simply put, there's no point having a goal that's totally unrealistic. For example, research suggests that not many men under 6ft/1.85m tall can reach 90kg in weight with body fat under 10%, so this wouldn't count as a realistic aim unless you're extremely gifted genetically, or are willing to take steroids (and let me make it clear here that I'm not advocating steroids at all: I never have and never will use them, but unfortunately over the years a lot of fitness/ physique models have encouraged otherwise unrealistic expectations). Keep your expectations realistic: it makes the process so much more enjoyable – especially when you finally reach your goal!

Timed

Timing your goals is very important, but the timing must be realistic. Setting realistic time scales will ensure you reach them, simply because you'll have something to aim for and it'll stop you putting goals off. Without any real pressure on you to train and improve you may let other things come between you and your goals. Furthermore, you won't get disheartened if you don't reach your goal in time, despite training as hard as you could. Set timed goals as realistically as possible, then even if the times have to be modified at least you've had something to work towards.

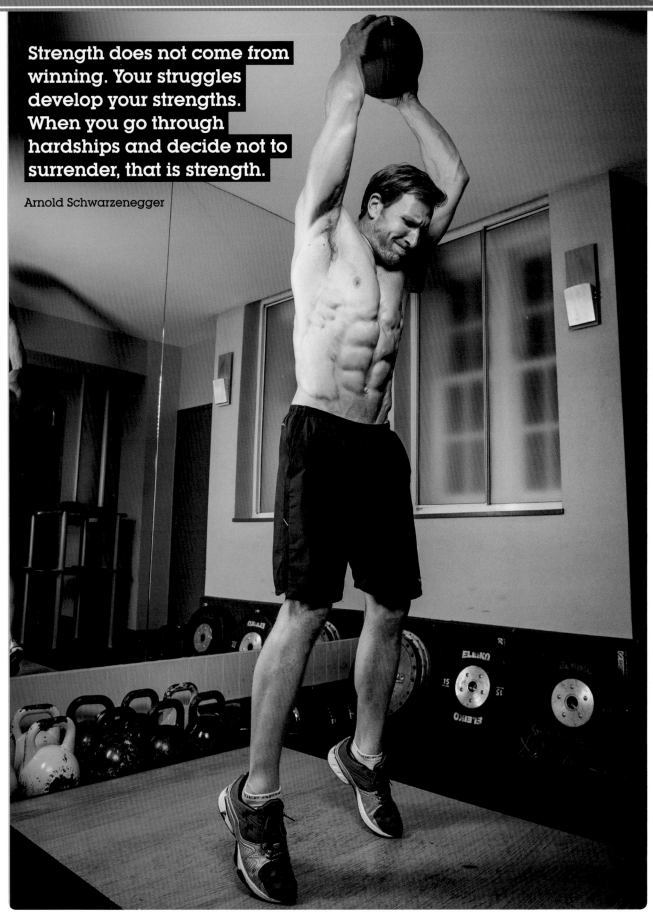

Strength does not come from winning. Your struggles develop your strengths. When you go through hardships and decide not to surrender, that is strength.

Arnold Schwarzenegger

A word on what's *really* possible

You have to be realistic in terms of your expectations regarding what's actually achievable without the use of drugs. It's fair to say that (some) poor personal trainers, gym chains, supplement brands and fitness magazines make unrealistic claims as to how much muscle you can add and how much fat you can lose in a short period of time. But you have to be realistic. Think about it: if it was easy to add muscle, then no one would need to take steroids or other drugs, and pretty much everyone would be walking around looking great. It's not the case! To look the way Hollywood suggests we should takes time, effort and money. Notice I said time first. The trick is to not fall foul of the unrealistic expectations that media, product manufacturers, gyms and some trainers have created to part you from your money. All that will happen is that you'll become disheartened, frustrated and ultimately give up when impossible goals over impossible timeframes aren't achieved.

Think of it this way. If you decided to take up triathlon today, having done very little running, swimming or cycling in your lifetime, would you expect to do a sub two-hour Olympic distance within the year? (Professionals complete the varying course between 1hr 40min and 1hr 50min depending on terrain.) It's not likely, is it? In fact, truth be told, its very unlikely *ever*. It takes years of training and a certain amount of good genetics to actually perform such an athletic feat. And gaining a large amount of muscle is actually the same. It takes time and real effort, not to mention the fact we don't all have the genetics to achieve high levels of natural muscle and remain Hollywood-lean naturally.

Take me, for example. I can hand-on-heart swear on family members' lives that I've never taken steroids, growth hormones or any other illegal substance to help build my physique. I still get asked if I have, I still have people disbelieving me when I state that I haven't. After all, I've been on national and international fitness covers, national fitness campaigns and BBC adverts, and earn money from my low-body-fat, muscular physique. What people don't know is that I was born in 1980. I first joined a gym (lying about my age) at 13 years old (having been doing press-ups and sit-ups from the age of 9 or 10 in the house). At school I played sports, ran or trained in the gym every day. At university I preferred to occupy the gym than the bar before, between and after lectures (as in my mind I was already preparing for my career as a Royal Marines officer). I

spent eight years as a Marine, exercising (give or take) every day, on many days doing two sessions: not just a little bit of exercise, but hard 'bootneck phys sessions'. I undertook multiple fitness-related courses and tests during my career and became a qualified Royal Marines Physical Training Instructor. Since leaving the Marines, I've pretty much trained for physique goals to allow me to earn money as a sports model, personal trainer, actor and fitness writer. It's my job.

From the above, you can ascertain that I've been completing harder and more intense training than most people almost daily, for around 20 years. Doesn't make my physique seem quite as unrealistic, does it? On top of that, I have parents and grandparents who were all very sporty, athletic and lean. My father was equivalent to what was back then a professional rugby player, and an English schools 100m champion, while my grandfather was a boxer and my mother an ice skater and sprinter. Utilising Malcolm Gladwell's arguments in his amazing book *Outliers*, I'm an outlier: I had all the right culminations of events in my life to allow me to have the physique I have today (though of course, I had to seize and act upon them). I was also born in September ... if you haven't read *Outliers* that won't make sense, so I suggest you read it. After this book, obviously.

What am I saying, then? That I was 'lucky', genetically, career-wise etc? No. What I'm trying to say is that despite my statement above about research suggesting it's near impossible for a male to naturally reach 90kg at a decent low-body-fat percentage unless they're over 185cm tall, it can be done. In general, I'd agree – especially if they're 23 or 24 years old, as many young physique models are. Where are *their* years of hard work? However, I'm only 182cm tall, yet I weigh 86kg and have body fat below 10% pretty much all the time (Christmas and birthdays are a given!).

Again, all I'm saying is that you have to be realistic. The young drug-fuelled physiques and unrealistic claims make everyone believe they can look like Ryan Reynolds. Equally, everyone thinks you can look like a cover model in three months. Well, from the hard work I've explained that I've put in, you'll realise that's actually rather unlikely for most people, unless they've already been training for some time. It takes time, hard work and dedication. Then it's far sweeter when you achieve your goal, and you'll look after your new body all the better too.

If it was easy, everyone would have a great body. If everyone had one, it would cease to be special, rare or desirable and nobody would want one any more.

If we take you today and only add muscle (but don't lose any fat) for three months, you'll still have a lower body fat percentage than when we started. Yes, even if we haven't actually lost any body fat. 'What?' I hear you cry. Well, think of it this way. Today you weigh 80kg and are 20% body fat, but in 12 weeks you'd be 83kg; but that 3kg is all added muscle. You'll therefore now have a lower body-fat percentage over your whole body, as more muscle has been added. Make sense? The problem is, you'll weigh more (which will freak out most of you, as scales seem to mean everything), despite your body-fat percentage decreasing due to simple maths. That's why my favourite tool for seeing if a transformation is working is the simple photograph. Take a picture once a day or once a week, front, side and back, and compare weekly.

Don't give up yet

Before I put you off completely, what can you really achieve over 12 weeks? Well, to start with, research suggests that a realistic rate of muscle gain for an absolute beginner is roughly 1kg per month. This figure is based around three things:

1 Good nutrition (not just content, but amounts and timings).
2 Intense training (something we'll speak about later) from a structured/planned resistance-based training programme (like the one in this book).
3 Average genetics (no need to be Hollywood perfect ... yet).

This means that you should only be able to put on 3kg of muscle during the 12 weeks, correct? Well, possibly not. If you're already training and/or have been in good shape previously but let it slip away, then research suggests you may be able to surpass the 1kg per month, due to your 'muscle memory' and the fact that your body is just regaining what it's previously had. You could (only could, note) gain more.

Let's assume it's around the 3kg mark for the 12-week period. That's pretty good going really. Remember, we aren't looking to build the next Mr Universe. (Ladies, pay attention – it's even harder for you to gain muscle: you don't have the testosterone the guys have.) What we want to do is lower your body fat and increase your muscle mass, and, bearing in mind that muscle weighs more than fat, if we end up with a lighter version of you (which is likely, unless you're a skinny ectomorph at this point who finds it hard to gain muscle), you would have not only gained 3kg of muscle but lost at least 3–4kg of fat, as you now weigh less. Now think of it this way: you want to look better (or 'toned' as you might like to call it), *ie* you want a body compositional change – basically a lower body-fat percentage. Well, if you weigh less and have more muscle, then the percentage of your body that will be made of fat will have gone down considerably.

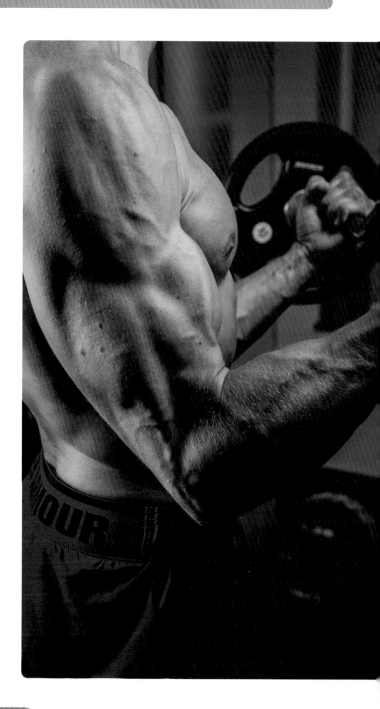

Time management: planning and training

The most difficult thing can be fitting the training in. Whether you currently go to the gym or not, chances are this programme will be asking more of you. Whether it's more trips to the gym, more sessions overall, or using your spare time to prepare your food, time management is crucial – especially when fitting in training with your working, sleeping, eating and family routine. It's tough; but it's not impossible.

Fitting in training

■ Just like a good job, training should be *part* of your life, not your *entire* life. Make sure you can see and recognise the difference.

■ In the everyday world, most people's lives revolve around a 9–5, five-day working week. Fitting training around this isn't actually that difficult. Just remember that it's a *part* of the day, not the main focus of the day. It's OK to look forward to it (or equally to dread it!), but make sure you also have time for your family and friends. Make sure you remain a well-rounded individual and don't become an obsessive.

■ 'I don't have time' is something I hear a lot when I write people training programmes or tell them what I need them to do in the seven days before I see them again. But making time is easy, as long as you're prepared to give up something else (TV programmes, football with the lads, shopping trip, nights out, Facebook...). It all comes down to how much you want it.

Working in time slots

Looking at the normal 9–5/8–6, generally five-day working week (*ie* with at least two days off per week), there are certain times that can easily be used for training. Yes, they may entail some extra organisation, they may even require you to get out of bed 30 minutes earlier to allow time to change and so on, but if you really want something then you'll do it. If you don't, you'll find an excuse. You need to have the commitment and dedication.

As I learned in the Marines, we humans give up in our minds long before our bodies fail. You can endure a lot of hardship for a few months, so a 12-week training programme where you're a little busier and get out of bed a little earlier (especially in the later stages) is nothing if it gets you that six-pack in time for your holiday.

Time slots
■ Before work
■ Lunchtime
■ Straight after work
■ Evenings
■ Weekends

Preparation is key

Preparing yourself is key to making this work. Make the time in the evening to pack your gym bag and prepare your food for the next day. Get everything ready, and make it a routine. That way you won't get to the gym to find you don't have any shorts ... bottomless training is banned at most gyms.

Training timings

Everyone is different and like to train at different times. If you can, get into a routine so that you know when you'll be training each day over your 12 weeks. Personally, I prefer to train my low intensity steady state (LISS) cardio early morning, before breakfast and work, and my resistance training or intervals mid-afternoon. However, I went through a long period where I couldn't train in the afternoon due to a course I was on, and therefore trained late morning. Again, it has to work with and around your lifestyle.

Despite me saying that, there are better times to train for your body to get the best results from this process. I wouldn't advise you to do your resistance training before work, for instance, as most people struggle to eat enough before the session. Therefore lunchtime or evening should be the norm, unless you're lucky enough to be able to take time out in the afternoon.

Lunchtime has long been a dividing line between co-workers (it's one of the busiest times in the gym). Half an office will sit at the desk eating or, if the weather's good, sit in the park; the other half will scoot to the gym to work out and shower in their hour off, before hitting the desk to scoff some food before restarting work. I used to do this in the Marines. I'd recommend it. You'll be surprised how much more productive you are after your session ... which may perhaps be a way to convince your boss to give you one hour 15 minutes to allow sufficient time for your session.

As for weekends, the programme in this book is structured to give you most of your weekends off, to rest and to do the other important things in your life. However, if you find it tough to train in the week, then you could shift the days around to train over the weekend instead – it's your life. Just consider the options and make it happen.

Lifestyle

Your life is your life. At the moment, you can probably write down how it plays out on a weekly basis, give or take. It has a pattern. We humans are very habitual. Chances are you set the alarm for the same time every morning, watch the same TV shows each week, go to the cinema or yoga or watch the football at the same time or place each week, and so on. We can't help it. That's how we work.

However, there are things that upset this balance. We create a nice, easy, sensible lifestyle, then things come along that force it to change: a new love interest, a baby, a new job, the death of a

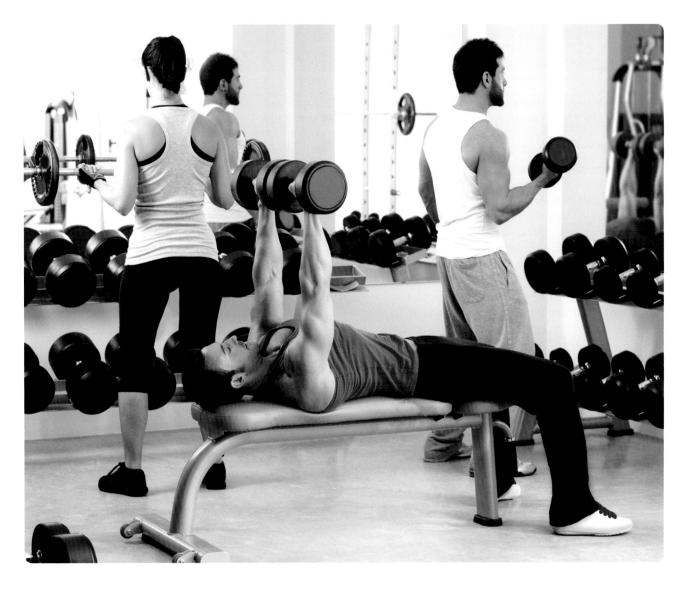

loved one, moving house etc. All pretty big, life-changing events, aren't they?

Well, guess what? If you let it, your body transformation can also be a life-changing event. I've had people who I've transformed come back and say to me: 'I can't thank you enough. My life, my goals, my focus is completely different. Thank you!' Take our cover model. After our transformation, he left his 9-5, packed his bags and moved to the Carribean with his fianceé. So, like all life-changing events, you have to be willing to change your lifestyle to accommodate it. If you don't want to, then stop now and do something else. Stay as you are, but learn to love what you have.

If you still wish to follow your plan, then be prepared to do WHATEVER it takes: stop smoking, stop drinking (yes, completely), give up caramel popcorn at the cinema, stop eating lunch with everyone at the High Street sandwich shop and above all, *above all*, ensure that you do your training every time it's scheduled. Bar life-threatening situations, training, like breathing, eating and sleeping, is one of your 'must dos', every day. At least for 12 weeks.

Circadian rhythms

Research suggests that humans have semi-regular sleep/wake cycles that attempt to follow the same pattern daily. These are called circadian rhythms. They supposedly regulate a huge number of our body's physiological functions, from blood pressure to metabolism. Studies indicate that our individual rhythms conform to our individual activities – daily alarm clock, meal times, bedtime and exercise times. They also demonstrate that we can teach our bodies to be 'good' at exercising at a certain time, by consistently exercising at that time.

Regularity seems to be the key for these rhythms. This doesn't mean that you can't train at different times, it just means that if you always train at a similar time, your body will be expecting it and therefore perhaps perform better. However, research also suggests that no matter when we think we're best suited to exercising, almost all of us are, in fact, physically stronger and have more endurance in the late afternoon, when we've fuelled our bodies for the day.

A fresh start

By failing to prepare, you are preparing to fail.

Benjamin Franklin

When I joined the Marines, they made it clear that our training (all 13 months of it) had to be our only priority in life. Men who attempted it with 'baggage' usually didn't make it. Yes, some people can compartmentalise, but most can't, and therefore need all their ducks in a row. Attempting your body transformation is very similar. You need to ensure that all those distractions are dealt with. If there's anything that can be put to bed in your life that'll otherwise just distract you on this journey, sort it now before you start. It'll only come back to distract you. Believe me, I've seen it in businessmen, students, single mothers, people from all walks of life. Put plans in place, get things sorted and finalised and *then* start the process. Otherwise you're setting yourself up for a fall.

Mental fitness

Mental fitness is something the majority of people don't even consider. However, mental fitness is often all that separates champions from the also-rans. Yes, some people are genetically gifted, but that doesn't mean anything if they don't have the right attitude to push themselves, work hard and achieve.

To join the Royal Marines, young men must pass the Potential Royal Marines Course (PRMC). These evaluate the candidates' potential, their potential to be trained to develop the Royal Marines' 'Strength of Mind'. Not every Marine is superfit, despite the fact they all have to pass the Commando tests to gain their green beret. However, they do all have incredible mental strength. It's during training that they develop this mental fitness. It's taught to them and developed without them even realising it.

You also need to develop a certain type of mental robustness to complete this programme. You need to be able to overcome tiredness, to be able to push to 15 reps instead of 12 when asked to do 12–15, just because you want to beat what you did last time. You need to want to pick the heavier weights, to want to fail at 12 pull-ups not 11. See what I'm saying? Even professional bodybuilders, despite using steroids to gain their impressive physiques, have incredible mental strength. Steroids don't make muscles just appear. They still require the training to be done. Pro bodybuilders have an incredible work ethic when training, and much of that can be attributed to mental fitness: an almost obsessive determination to endure the discomfort and pain to reap the rewards.

Speaking of the Royal Marines, I think the Commando Values and Commando Spirit fit well here as things for you to think about over the next 12 weeks as you complete your body transformation:

The Commando Values

- Excellence – strive to do better. That's the point of the whole process, but take that into each session and try to beat what you did last time.
- Integrity – tell the truth. To yourself. Did you really work hard enough – as hard as you could?
- Self-discipline – resist the easy option. This is possibly the most important. Push to the limits each time. If you stop to rest, that set is done. You can't get it back.
- Humility – respect the rights, diversity and contribution of others. We'll come on to gym etiquette later, but these values obviously go hand in hand. Also, if you start to look good, remember where you came from. Don't be one of those bigheads.

The Commando Spirit

- Courage – get out front and do what's right, for you and for everyone around you. Do what's necessary and don't ever be afraid to fail.
- Determination – never give up. I don't need to add to this.
- Unselfishness – partner first, team second, self last. This works slightly differently in terms of a transformation. You have to be a little selfish to get it done, to make time for the training, food prep etc. But outside of that, try to be unselfish in your life. You'll feel good for it.
- Cheerfulness – make humour the heart of your morale. When things go wrong, try to laugh at it. When the pain of training really kicks in, try to laugh. It works. Keep your favourite joke or comedy film moment in mind and think of it when things get rough. It could always be worse...

Medical advice

Every fitness professional is taught to advise and suggest that anyone beginning any exercise programme who hasn't exercised for some time should consult a doctor beforehand. When training people, I always ask them if they've consulted their doctor and if there is any reason they shouldn't be exercising. Old injuries and operations, current medication, family traits, possibility of pregnancy and any medication being taken should

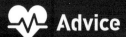

Advice

If you're new to exercise or returning after a good amount of time off, consult a doctor before you start. Just to be sure.

all have to be considered. Life's too short and too precious, so safety must always come first. It'll actually give you more confidence if you know that your body is healthy and able to undertake and complete what you're about to ask of it.

Kit and equipment

Before you start training you need to get yourself a few bits of kit. There are a number of things in this book that are personal and up to you. However, I believe you need all of the following to make your life easier and ensure you stick to your programme:

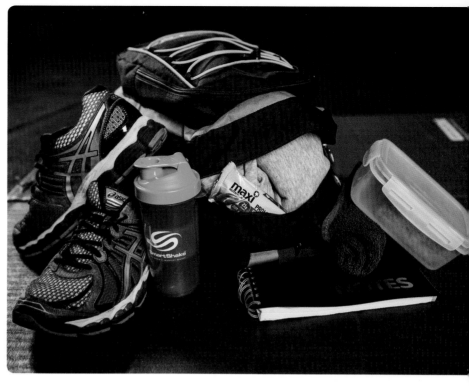

- Two or three sets of shorts and T-shirts to train in.
- A good pair of training shoes. Some people have a running pair and a lifting pair. I do. Squash, skateboard or football shoes are *not* acceptable.
- A water bottle.
- A shaker (or two). I recommend SmartShake.
- A stopwatch (or smartphone stopwatch).
- A notebook or smartphone logging app or training diary.
- A sweat towel and a normal towel.
- A digital camera or smartphone camera.
- Three of four Tupperware containers. I recommend Systema.
- Wrist straps or chalk.
- A sense of humour.

In the Royal Marines, we were also taught the following in relation to our kit:

- Look after your kit and your kit will look after you.
- Your weapon, your kit, your self.

The first is simple: whether it's your notebook, digital camera or shaker, look after it just the same. Your camera may be ten times the value of the other items, but it makes no difference, look after each of them properly. This means washing your shaker properly after every use. It'll stop it smelling and make it last longer. At the end of the day, it's for your comfort. I had one client who washed his shaker in the shower or sink after every session before he even left the gym. 'Good drills,' as we said in the Marines. However you do it, clean it and look after it.

This also goes for washing your kit. Never (NEVER) use the same set of gym kit twice without washing it. Even if you can't smell it, it smells. I often come into contact with people (99% of the time men) who blatantly haven't washed their kit. If it's a client, and they smell, they go home and I still get paid. Simple. I'm not breathing in that sweet, stale sweat smell for an hour. If

it's in a communal gym, then I avoid that person like the plague. If they keep coming near me, I explain to them one of the gym etiquette rules: it's a shared environment, so 'do unto others as you would like them to do unto you'. Wipe the bench, put kit back and wash your clothes after every use.

Preparation is key

Before you rush into training, read this book. It's not long, so read it, front to back. Don't pick through it, don't skip bits. Read it. All of it. Not for my benefit – once I've written it, that's my bit done – but for your own. If you read the whole thing then you won't miss anything: you won't start without sorting your nutrition (the biggest mistake you could make); you won't start and decide to skip the weekly photos or the training diary. You see where I'm coming from?

Everything that's taught to a Marine recruit in training is necessary. Nothing is included for fun. It's there for a reason. Those reasons aren't always apparent immediately, but there is a reason. This book is the same. I've approached it from that point of view, that style of training. So, take everything on board. In my opinion you should read this book right through, then, with a notepad and pen, plan your 12 weeks. If you have a weekend away, or family birthday or work trip, you need to plan around it now. Look at your work and social schedule: when's best for you to train? Days of the week, time of day and so on. Plan it all *now*.

Time spent rehearsing is seldom wasted. That's another Marine-ism. There'll be a few ... er, hundred more, but I believe my training was paramount to who I am today and what I can pass on to you I will. So take heed: take the time to plan your next 12 weeks. Things may change, but at least you'll be ready!

Marked progress

You need to make sure you can see what changes are occurring, so to do this you need to take measurements at the start and throughout the programme. I advise the following measurements to be taken. However, I'm going to suggest you weigh yourself I don't believe that weight is a good indicator during a transformation, because, as we've already seen, muscle weighs more than fat. Thus a good 'body compositional change' will see your fat decrease and muscle increase, meaning you could weigh the same or actually more by the end of the 12 weeks.

Photographs

Use a digital camera to take the following pictures in as little clothing as you can (underwear/swimwear is best):

- Front.
- Back.
- Left side.
- Right side.

Take the first set of pictures on the Sunday evening before your first Monday session, then repeat this every week. Try to take the photos in the same place at the same time, in the same clothes. Keep the lighting the same as well if you can.

Measurements

Using a tape measure, measure the following areas. If you have a friend or partner (training or personal), get them to help you to ensure correct measurements are taken:

- Chest (over nipple area for men, under breasts for women).
- Shoulders (just below bony area).
- Arms (with arm bent, so biceps flexed).
- Stomach (around belly button).
- Thighs (the point halfway between hip and knee).
- Hips (around widest point).

Be as accurate as possible and write down all the measurements with the date you took them. Repeat every week, every two weeks or monthly.

Note that some people advise measuring down, up or across from certain points on the body and marking those points with a pen, then taking the measurements at those points to ensure they're always taken at exactly the same spots. Bony nodules, the belly button, moles and so on are good places to measure from. This isn't absolutely necessary, but it can help.

Weight

As I said, this is my least favourite method of seeing progress, yet it seems to be everyone's obsession! To give you an idea of why I disapprove, I'm now in the high 80s in terms of my weight in kilograms, whereas when I was in the Marines I weighed 78–80kg, yet my body fat was higher. I now have more muscle but weigh more and look leaner. See my point?

Weigh yourself at the same time of day each time and always use the same scales. Obviously, ensure you're wearing little to nothing and the same each time.

Learning

Everyone learns differently. This has been studied and researched, and that's the only real conclusion. There are a number of different thought processes as to how we learn and the different ways. However, I'm going to give just one, possibly the most well-known and simplest – Neil Fleming's VAK/VARK model:

- Visual learners.
- Auditory learners.
- Reading-writing preference learners.
- Kinaesthetic learners or tactile learners.

Visual learners have a preference for seeing pictures, visual aids, diagrams and demonstrations. Auditory learners need to listen to lectures and discussions. Reading/writing learners ... well, that's

simple: reading a book such as this and making their own notes. Finally, kinaesthetic/tactile learners prefer to learn via experience, by actually doing the thing being taught and experimenting.

Unfortunately, I only have this book to pass on the information I need to. That may not suit you and your learning style unless you're a reader/writer, but what choice do we have?

This brings me to the one phrase that has appeared in all my books: know thyself. What I mean by this is that you need to look at yourself. Step back and take a look. What drives you? Why did you buy this book? What makes you want to read this book? More importantly, what will stop you reading it? What will prevent you from fulfilling the goal that has driven you to buy this book in the first place? If you get to the bottom of that one you'll succeed, not just in this, but in life.

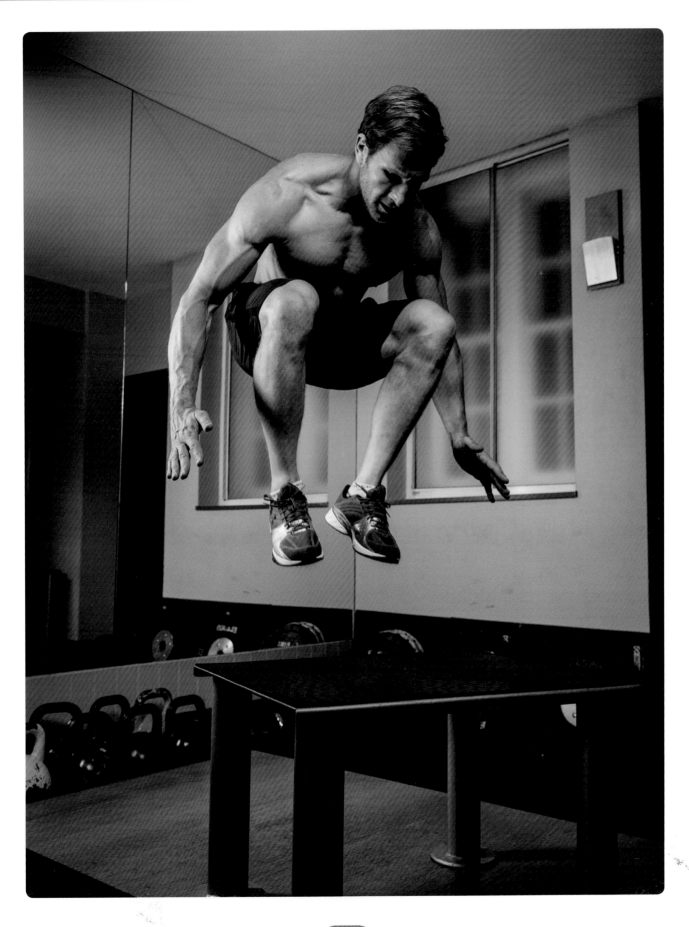

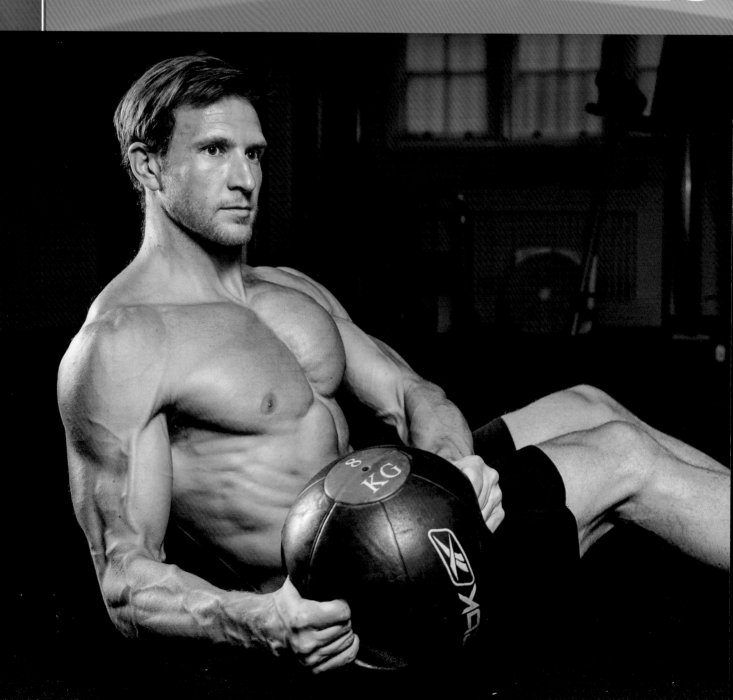

CHAPTER 3
EXERCISE FUNDAMENTALS

Although this book is designed to be something you can read from front to back and then simply follow the guidelines and training programme to reap the benefits, I'm a big fan of also imparting knowledge and information. This chapter therefore explains a few exercise fundamentals that should help you see why we do what we're going to do and, equally perhaps, why you should stop doing what you used to do!

Exercise types

Compound exercises

Compound exercises work several muscle groups at the same time and include movement around two or more joints. The main examples are:

- Squat.
- Deadlift.
- Overhead press.
- Bench press.
- Pull-up/Lat pull down

These are often the main five exercises that a strength programme is based around, as they hit all the muscles around all the joints between them. They include movements around multiple joints like the shoulder and elbow or hip, knee and ankle.

Compound exercises are the ones that any good training programme should start with and centre around for the duration, as they burn more calories due to involving more and larger muscles. Free weights and callisthenics are my preference for compound movements, though some machines like the leg press and lat pulldown have their place.

Isolation exercises

Isolation exercises are those that only exercise one joint. Examples include the biceps curl, leg curl and leg extension. Although isolation exercises can be performed with some joints using free weights, like the biceps curl or triceps extension, to exercise the quadriceps of the legs requires a leg extension machine, to ensure that other muscle groups are minimally involved and to ensure a stable posture.

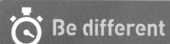 **Be different**

To change you, you must progress your gym training. If your training is the same week in week out – same weights, same exercises, same sessions – then you'll also remain the same.

In short, compound exercises should be favoured to isolation during sessions. However, isolation exercises can be used to great effect to keep the heart rate up after a compound exercise or at the end of a session, to further fatigue single muscles. Isolation exercises are also required for bringing up certain muscles to help the overall aesthetic look of a physique.

Progression

Progression is what it says on the tin: progressing. It's what we're told from a young age we should be doing; progressing from liquid to solid food, from primary school to secondary, from education to employment, from single to being in a relationship, from renter to homeowner. The list goes on. Life is all about improving and progressing, and your body compositional change is no different. You have to progress. The way to progress is to work harder and change the variables within a session. If you don't progress, you won't change as much as you could, so put the effort in and force change by forcing progression.

Variables

Variables are the things we can change. In science, we come up with a hypothesis and then change a variable to see if it gives us results that support the hypothesis. The other variables are kept constant. To progress your training and force your body to change and adapt to stimuli created in your sessions, the variables MUST be changed. One or more of the variables can be changed – it doesn't have to be one alone, although changing a number of them can make the session increasingly more intense than before. Although progression is necessary and intensity is key to change and reaching your goal, going too hard too soon can result in you giving up or getting injured, so tread carefully and be sensible. The following are a list of variables that can be changed:

- Frequency of sessions: At first this is likely to be three to four sessions a week, but it can increase up to six.
- Number of sessions: You'll start out with one session a day, but two sessions can be performed if necessary. These can be one cardiovascular and one resistance, or two resistance. If doing two, try to ensure a time period of at least four hours between them; six or more is preferable.
- Type of session: LISS (low intensity steady state) cardiovascular sessions can be made more intense and progressed by changing them to HIIT (high intensity interval training) sessions. Simple standard set hypertrophy sessions can become supersets, trisets or giant sets (see below), all progressing the session.
- Weight used in the session: The weight can be increased each session, making the body work harder to reach the reps required. However, increase weight sensibly. If you can't lift it fully or properly, then the increased weight won't progress you, as you aren't training properly.
- Timing of session: The session can last 20 minutes or up to 75 minutes. A 10-minute HIIT session can be progressed rapidly if it lasts 20 minutes the next time.
- Sets of an exercise: Increasing from three sets to four, five or even, in the case of GVT (German volume training), ten. Obviously, increasing sets progresses that exercise and the associated muscles drastically.

- Reps of an exercise: Reps can be increased or decreased to force progression and change. However, a decrease in reps should see an increase in weight to match and still ensure intensity (see opposite). Lowering reps but using the same weight won't give adequate training stimulus unless rest time is greatly reduced.
- Rest timings of session: The amount of rest has a huge effect on the muscles and the session. Keeping other variables constant yet dropping rest from 90 seconds to 30 will have huge effects on intensity. However, reducing rest often means weight/reps must be reduced.
- Tempo used for an exercise: Lifting and lowering a weight over just one second is far easier than lowering a weight over three seconds. Equally, taking a one-second pause at the top to recoup before starting the next rep makes the exercise easier compared to zero rest and starting the next rep immediately. Changing the tempo is a great way to progress an exercise or session and my personal 'go to' when someone asks me how to better their training. Most people just move the weight; they don't consider how they're moving it. Even a simple press up, done using a 4010 tempo (4 down, 0 hold at bottom, 1 up, 0 hold at top), becomes really hard very quickly.
- Training protocols used in session: Drop sets, rest/pause sets, forced reps, partial reps etc (see below). Utilising and changing these protocols within sessions has a huge effect on intensity, thus forcing the body to change – especially as the body can become accustomed to one and then need another one in order to progress.

Variables must take into account other variables when you manipulate them. Changing the weight, number of reps, protocol and tempo to make them all harder, plus reducing your rest, will see you regretting messing with so much all at once, and having to change everything as the session is now too hard. Change just one or maybe two at a time (in terms of making one harder and another easier to make the goal feasible). Always be realistic, and open to compromise if you've made things too tough!

 Variety is key

Without variation you become stagnant. When asked, 'What's the best exercise/protocol for...', respected exercise physiologist and nutritionist Jim Stoppani PhD says, 'The one you aren't doing.' The message? Change regularly to keep the body guessing and changing.

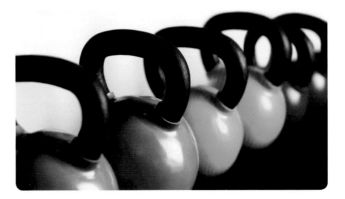

Intensity

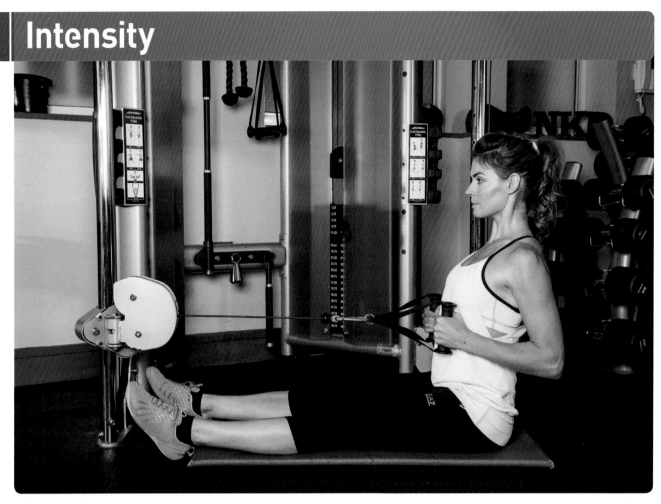

Intensity is probably the single most important thing for someone to get right when training. It's also the one thing that most people believe they get right. However, they're usually way off.

OK, arguably nutrition is more important. However, if I'm going to be honest, I'd rather someone transformed their body using exercise and healthy eating than just diet alone: someone could just make sure they're in a calorific deficit day to day and carry on with life as normal, and as long as they don't veer too far from the way they should be eating for their calorific deficit, they'll lose weight (not necessarily fat, though). However, although this nutritional change will see them lose weight, they won't gain muscle (the metabolic tissue we need to see positive lifelong changes); and without muscle gain, when they eventually fall off their diet wagon they'll add weight again (in the form of body fat). Why? Because they'll inevitably eat the things they

like or want and be in a calorific surplus. If they're unlucky, all that dieting without exercise will also cause their metabolic rate to slow a bit, meaning they can take even less calories. Again, when they come off their diet they'll put the weight back on. Isn't that the story you hear from most people who diet without training? In fact even those that diet and train 'a bit' (jogging and cardio-based LISS exercise mainly) say the same; they bounce back bigger if they go back to more 'normal' eating habits once they've lost some weight.

So what's the answer? If dieting/nutritional change alone isn't the answer, and dieting/nutritional change with cardiovascular training isn't the answer, what is? Simple: intense resistance training teamed with LISS and/or HIIT training and a sensible calorific deficit.

They key word here is INTENSE. Your training has to be

The last three or four reps is what makes the muscle grow. This area of pain divides the champion from someone else who is not a champion. That's what most people lack, having the guts to go on and just say they'll go through the pain no matter what happens.

Arnold Schwarzenegger

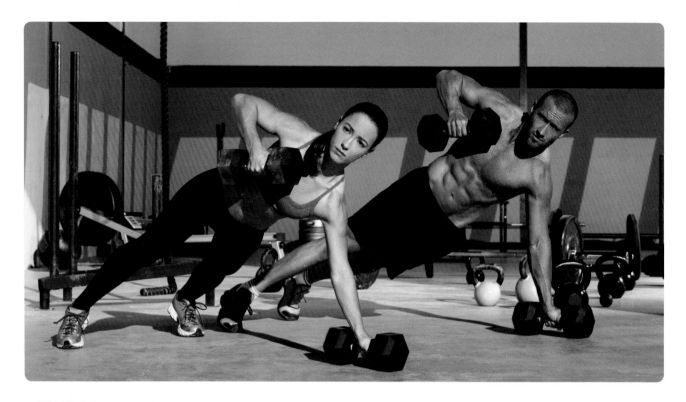

Nothing in the world is worth having or worth doing unless it means effort, pain, difficulty.

Theodore Roosevelt

intense. If it's easily achievable, it isn't intense. If you aren't sweating, it isn't intense. If you could carry on for another 30 minutes, it isn't intense. If you can stand there texting or tweeting between sets, it isn't intense. If you could do another ten reps with that weight after doing your desired reps range, it isn't intense. If you can go back to work or go home without

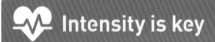

Intensity is key

Without intensity your sessions are no better than a slow jog around the park. They'll raise your heart rate, burn a few calories, but won't help you progress past the point you are at.

showering following your session (which you should NEVER do), it isn't intense. Make sense?

One of my favourite slogans is 'Intensity is key'. If you train with intensity, each set should be close to failure. Each interval should have you itching to finish. Every session should give you that little butterfly of nerves in your stomach. Once you have that, you're training hard. You'll probably often feel a little sick during your sessions, but you'll have the body you want in no time at all. Training with a partner or trainer can help with intensity, as humans naturally, unconsciously will choose the safer, easier option. Well, don't. And if you have a training partner, help them push harder and progress (sensibly and safely).

Failure

Failure goes hand in hand with intensity. It's a way to make the session intense, and it's what each of the progressions mentioned above is trying to get you to. You increase the weight, up the reps, lower the rest etc, to get to a point where you can't do what it is you're *trying* to do. It sounds counter-intuitive, but it's a simple fact. It needs to be the way you train. It makes a stimulus to which your body needs to adapt, so that the changes you want occur: increased muscle, lower body fat (due to calorific deficit) and, soon enough, a body compositional change.

Just like in bodybuilding, failure is also a necessary experience for growth in our own lives, for if we're never tested to our limits, how will we know how strong we really are? How will we ever grow?

Arnold Schwarzenegger

Time under tension

Tension is one of the most important factors for inducing hypertrophy (muscle enlargement). Tension is created when our muscles contract against a heavy load. The fibres of the muscle have to work against the weight, and that tension triggers a series of reactions in the body. Simply put, adding tension to the muscles causes a cascade of chemical reactions that lead to increased protein synthesis in the fibres. As we know, though, if we don't get enough protein, and food in general, these reactions can still be wasted.

To be a bit more scientific, the regulator of muscle protein synthesis is the 'mTOR pathway', mTOR standing for 'mammalian target of rapamycin'. Don't worry, you don't need to understand the science; only that research has shown that the more mTOR is stimulated in your body, the more protein synthesis occurs, and that there's a direct relationship between mTOR and tension: the more tension a muscle is put under, the greater the mTOR stimulation.

There are two types of tension to consider:

1. Load.
2. Time under tension (TUT).

The larger the weight lifted, the more increased the tension. This in turn stimulates mTOR more, thereby increasing protein synthesis at a higher level, which is what makes the muscles grow. If you think about it, that's just one of our variables to ensure intensity, isn't it? Increasing the weight. So as long as we lift heavier and heavier weights, keeping the intensity high, this will build more muscle and in turn lower body fat through hard training and sensible nutrition.

Not quite...

It's not just about the direct tension placed on the muscle from a heavy weight. The time the muscle is under tension is really important. Hence TUT. TUT also stimulates regulation of the mTOR pathway, meaning the longer the muscles are under tension, the more protein synthesis is increased. Simple then: to increase TUT, lifting a lighter weight with a really slow tempo while still maintaining good form and a sensible nutritional plan will provide the best increases in protein synthesis. Well, almost. If the weight is too light, mTOR won't be triggered. Equally, research suggests that it actually switches off after around 60 seconds of tension. Thus there's an optimum balance of load and TUT.

Still with me? Put it this way: picking the heaviest weight, if you can do only one good rep with perfect form it'll provide a massive amount of tension, but will lack TUT. The set will be over in 3–5 seconds max. The trick is to find the heaviest weights that can be lifted for a little under 60 seconds.

In this programme we'll be using tempo (point 9 in the list on page 26). This indicates the timings of the various stages of the lift. You'll generally be using 3010 or 4010. Either way, one rep takes 3–5 seconds (1 second up, 0 second hold, 3/4 seconds down, 0 seconds at the bottom). We'll then be working at rep ranges of 5–15 reps depending on the microcycle chosen. This rep range, combined with the given tempo, should maximise both the load and the TUT.

As I've said, variation is key to stopping the body's adaption to a given demand, which is why we're going to change the reps ranges and weight; so although people like to argue whether 8 reps is better than 15 reps for muscle growth, in short it might not even matter, because the two factors (load and TUT), when combined equally with the correct weight and tempo, will basically give the same results anyway.

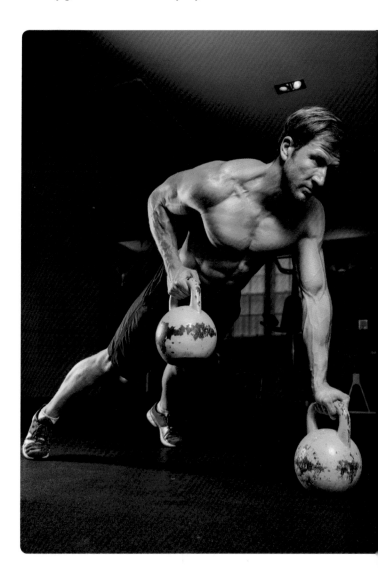

Legs

Simply put: training your legs is paramount.

Ladies' legs

Let's start with the girls for once, as actually you'll prefer training legs more than the boys, and probably prefer legs to upper body. So, ladies, if you train your legs with squats, deadlifts, lunges, split squats, step-ups and the like, you'll develop:

- A lovely set of legs.
- A pert bottom.

... and you'll start to look great in leggings, skirts and tight trousers (not to mention a bikini).

To reiterate what I said earlier, Victoria's Secret models perform squats, lunges, deadlifts etc, and do far more of this than running or cardiovascular training. They do these exercises to ensure they have a sexy, shapely figure so that they look good in underwear.

The weights exercises also have a better effect at lowering their body fat and allow them to eat more of the foods they like, because any extra muscle (metabolic tissue) they build helps them increase their metabolism.

However, those weights sessions need to be both intense and progressive (see the previous pages). If you're just doing sets of 30 reps without getting to the failure point, you may as well be jogging uphill. You're just doing cardiovascular training (after all, cardio training is just very low weight resistance training for long periods of time). You need to lift relatively heavy weights that make you struggle for 8–15 reps. When I say struggle, it needs to get you to a point where you start to fail and need to put the weight down between 8 and 15 reps. Rest for your specified time, then do the next set, again trying to hit failure point.

But, ladies, legs aren't everything. You still need to do upper body training to ensure shapely arms and shoulders; and again, the weights need to be meaningful, and the sessions intense!

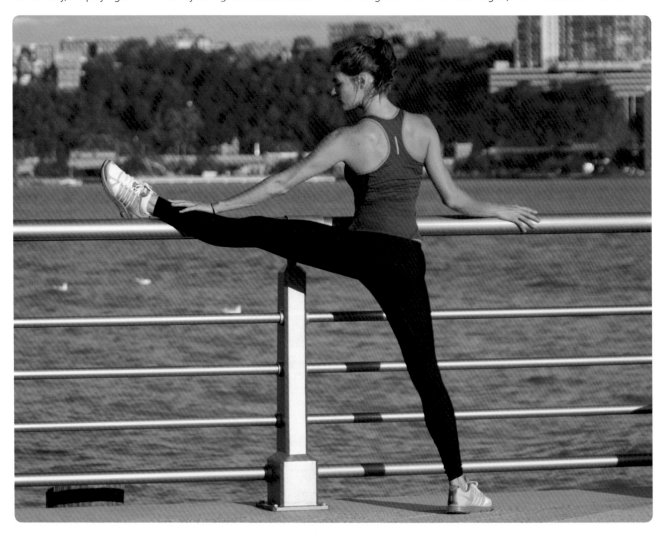

Guys' legs

Have you seen those guys in the gym who have skinny legs but great big upper bodies? They look stupid, don't they? Many will have taken steroids, to allow their upper bodies to grow while their legs haven't. You don't want to look like that and you don't want to be one of those guys with big upper and no lower.

The answer? Train your legs – not as an afterthought, but as your main session every week. In fact, legs should be trained twice a week, or at least every 5/6 days. I appreciate that your 'beach weights' or 'mirror muscles' (pecs, abs, biceps and shoulders) are far more important to you, but you don't want half the package. You don't want to end up as one of those guys who ALWAYS wears tracksuit bottoms in the gym to hide their legs, because you'll eventually have to hit the beach or pool on holiday and show those little toothpicks, and the bigger your upper body is, the smaller they'll look.

Still not convinced? What If I told you that training legs will help your upper body grow? Burn more calories both in the session and by building the largest muscles in your body, increase your metabolism allowing you to eat more of the

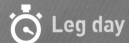

Leg day

Leg day is arguably the most important session of your training programme. It has so many physiological advantages, not to mention crafting an attractive set of legs for both sexes.

things you like, while helping to help you keep your body fat lower so you can see your abs? Also, most leg exercises with free weights require so much core stability that they'll give you a better six-pack than the endless sit-ups you're doing. Starting to get the picture? Let me completely convince you: your body responds to the larger weights you lift when training squats and deadlifts by upping the levels of testosterone and growth hormone your body produces, not to mention the mTOR pathway protein synthesis explained on page 29. Lifting these heavy weights when doing these exercises will actually help you grow those pecs, biceps, delts, lats and traps you crave so badly. It's that simple. *Never* skip a leg session (unless injured of course).

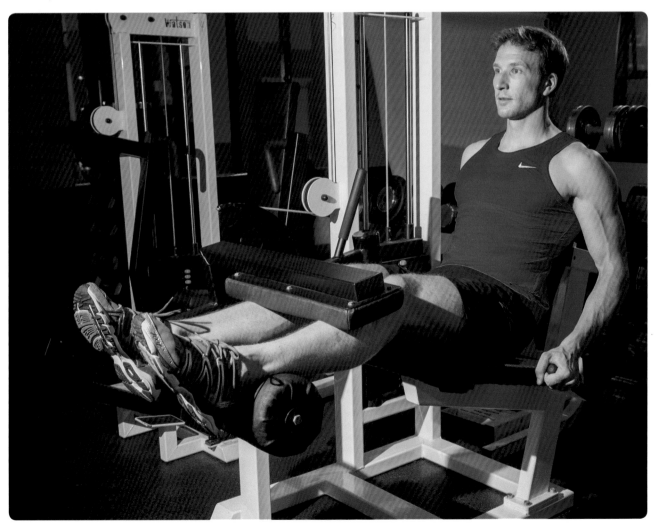

Training partners

I've personally trained alone, with other Marines, with friends, with my girlfriend and with clients. As a trainer, I've trained people who've never trained with a partner, those who have, and those who've never trained with a trainer before. What I've found with all of them is that even the most focused, self-believing, driven people struggle to train to the same level alone. That's why people pay personal trainers – not just to write them a programme and diet plan, but to stand there and motivate them to work hard, push through failure and stimulate the body's changes faster than if they trained alone.

Working with a training partner is something you should try to do. When you're having a bad day (lack of sleep, work getting you down, social life has taken a downward spiral) your training partner will help you. Conversely, you'll repay them on another day when the tables have turned. However, more important than that, you'll push each other and increase the session intensity simply by a little healthy competition. If the training programme says 12–15 reps and it starts hurting at 12, you'd probably stop if you were alone. But like a trainer, your partner is behind you (they haven't felt how tough it is yet) and encourages you to do 13, 14 or even 15. You've already surpassed what you'd have done on your own. Then your partner will get in there and do 15, because they can't let you down. You've both surpassed what you'd have done individually. Your partner will also ensure you do everything properly – they don't want you doing half reps, because they're going to do it properly, so you'd better too.

Everything becomes easier when training with someone – except the training!

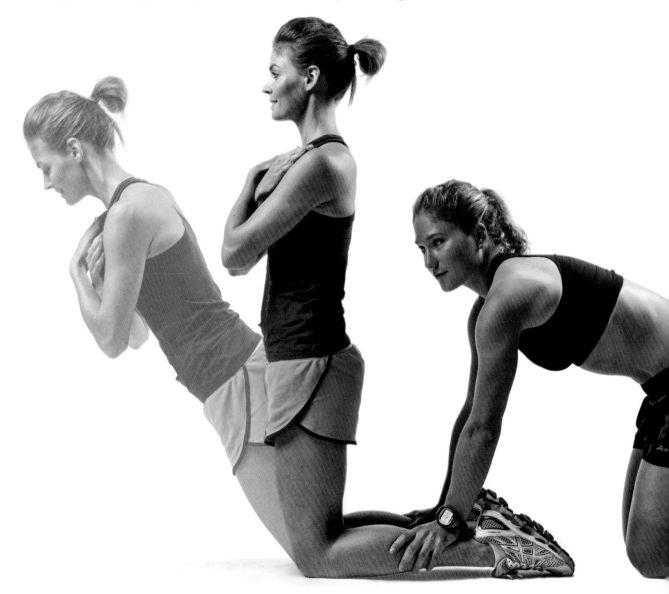

Training protocols

There are many different 'training protocols', each with the same basic principle behind them: to make you work more intensely, and thus force your muscles to change. Many of these protocols aim to induce muscle failure, which will spur the muscle to adapt and grow. Examples worth mentioning are:

Drop sets

Drop sets involve finishing your normal set, then dropping the weight used by 20–30% and performing (up to) the same amount of reps as performed in the original set. Two drops are usually performed, which would mean again dropping the weight by 20–30% before performing the third set.

Rest/pause sets

Similar to drop sets, in that two further sets are usually performed rather than just one. After the first set rest for 10–15 seconds, then perform as many more reps as you can with the same weight. Rest again for 10–15 seconds and again perform as many reps as possible with the same weight again. 10, 6 and 4 are good numbers to aim for if you're using a weight for 10–12 reps.

Partial reps

Partial reps involve performing your set to the point of failure with full reps, using as near to perfect technique as you can. However, once you fail it's possible to perform partial reps in the easier area of the exercise. Every exercise has a 'sticking point' – the area where it's harder (the lowest part of a squat, bench press or pull-up would be good examples). So, as no more full reps can be performed, partial reps are accepted for a further few reps to take the muscles past failure.

Forced reps

Forced reps involve getting to the same place as above – failure – but instead of performing partials you perform full reps with a training partner helping you through the sticking point. This forces a few more reps and the muscles to adapt to that stimulus, increasing strength, endurance and hypertrophy over time.

Unilateral assistance

Unilateral assistance allows really heavy eccentric lowers (tempos like 4010) if you don't have a partner to help with forced reps. The basic idea is to focus on one limb at a time and use the maximal weight for that side. Use both limbs to lift the weight,

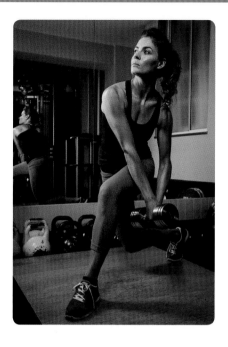

but only one to lower. Only use the 'assistance limb' as much as required to raise the weight.

Supersets

Supersets involve putting two exercises back to back for opposing muscle groups, for example bench press/chin-ups or biceps curls/triceps extension. The idea is to perform both exercises without rest, then rest between the supersets. Supersets can be made more intense by any of the other protocols above.

Compound sets

Similar to supersets, but instead of opposing muscle groups we use two exercises for the same muscle group, for example bench press and pec flyes or overhead press and lateral raise. It's always best to perform the larger/compound exercise first, *ie* the exercise involving more weight. Again, other protocols can be utilised with a compound set.

Trisets

Trisets are basically compound sets of three exercises instead of two, for example overhead press, upright row, lateral raise. As for compound sets, it's best to perform the heaviest/compound set first and move through the exercises in terms of weight and size/number of muscles exercised.

Giant sets

Giant sets are the same as trisets but with four or more exercises performed back to back without rest.

Session length

Each session should be no more than 45–60 minutes due to energy levels dropping, cortisol levels increasing, causing the body to want to store fat rather than burn it, and testosterone levels dropping – which is not good, as testosterone is paramount for muscle building.

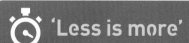

⏱ 'Less is more'

In the gym, the mantra 'Less is more' is often very true. Train hard and intense, but get in and get out. After all, you need to eat, sleep and prepare for tomorrow!

Making your body transform

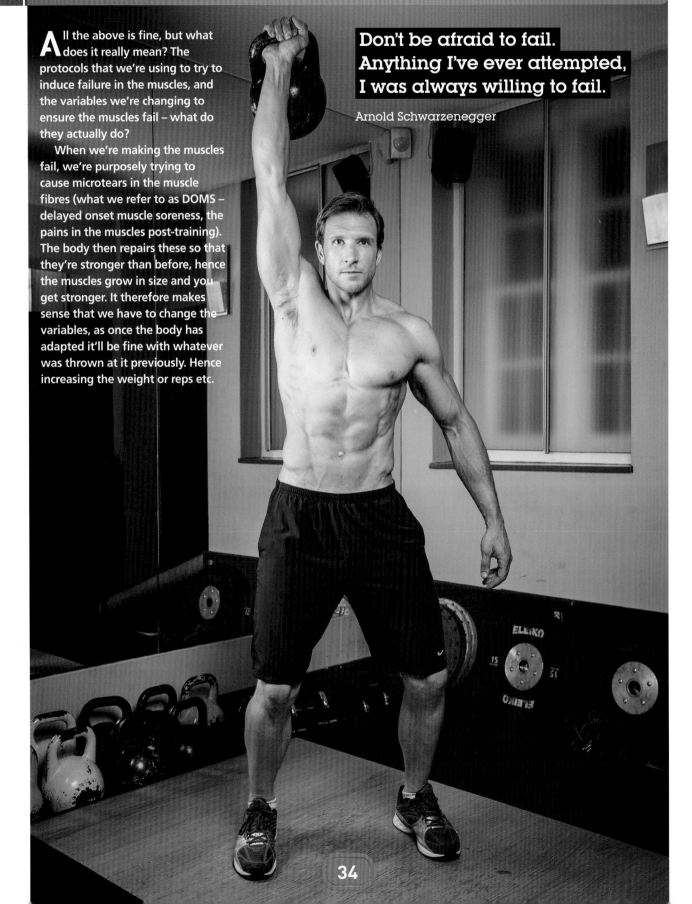

All the above is fine, but what does it really mean? The protocols that we're using to try to induce failure in the muscles, and the variables we're changing to ensure the muscles fail – what do they actually do?

When we're making the muscles fail, we're purposely trying to cause microtears in the muscle fibres (what we refer to as DOMS – delayed onset muscle soreness, the pains in the muscles post-training). The body then repairs these so that they're stronger than before, hence the muscles grow in size and you get stronger. It therefore makes sense that we have to change the variables, as once the body has adapted it'll be fine with whatever was thrown at it previously. Hence increasing the weight or reps etc.

Don't be afraid to fail. Anything I've ever attempted, I was always willing to fail.

Arnold Schwarzenegger

Rest

Rest is needed. Without rest you can't complete the training sessions or the programme. Whether we're discussing rest between sets or rest days between sessions, you have to listen to your body and rest – without being over-generous and losing the focus of your session.

For example, some of your sessions will require 60 seconds' rest between sets. If you're in a rush and only want to take 30 seconds, chances are you won't be able to lift the required weight for the required reps for all the sets. Yes, there'll be days where you're too rushed, so you'll need to tweak the sessions, but in general there are other things that can give way. As was said at the beginning of this book, if you can't focus on this process 100%, then wait until you're at a point in your life when you can.

Conversely, if you aren't feeling great, didn't sleep well or have low energy levels, you may need to up a 60-second rest to 75 seconds instead. Sometimes this is necessary to get the best out of the training, especially during drop sets or rest pauses sets. Having said that, try not to – try to work through it. Again, this is where a training partner can help. If they can do it, you can, and you won't want to let them down. Despite saying that, listen to your body; if you really

 Be uncomfortable

Like Royal Marine training, I believe you can never be in your comfort zone in the gym. If you are, you're coasting, and your muscles are finding the session too easy. Tweak one of the variables – tempo, weight, rest etc – or add a drop set or rest/pause set and make sure you work to that failure point to make the changes you want happen. The only person who loses out when you take it easy is you. You can never get a session back. Treat each session like it's your last.

are getting unwell or sick, then take a longer rest but still try to complete the session.

REST: recovery equals successful training

Yes, it may be a little silly, but the acronym 'REST' will help you remember why it's necessary to take time off and not overtrain. Take your rest days; they're in the programme for a reason.

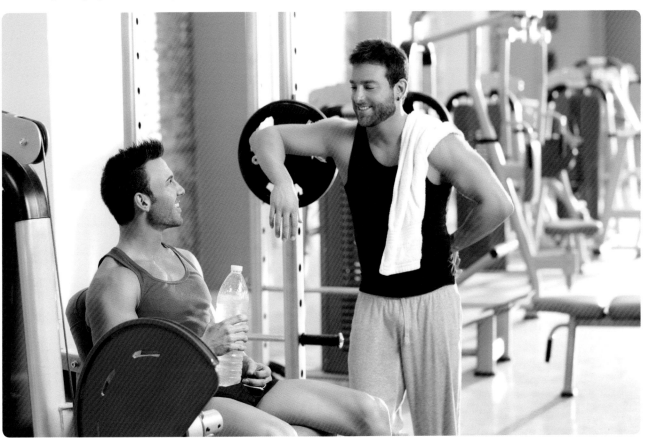

Warming up and cooling down

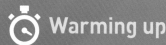

Warming up

If you haven't got time to warm up, then you haven't got time to train.

Why warm up?

It's imperative that you spend a few minutes at the beginning of each session warming up. Besides the obvious reason that it can help you avoid injury, the warm-up has many other benefits:

- It prepares the body for the session to come.
- It thoroughly warms the muscles, ligaments and tendons.
- It increases the core temperature of the body.
- It aids mental focus and prepares the mind for the session to come.
- It helps the neuromuscular channels prior to the session.

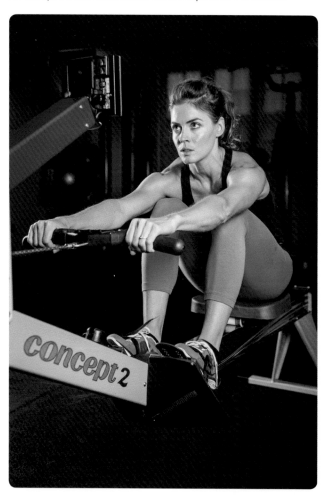

How long should you warm up?

There's no real set time for a warm-up; its length varies depending on its aim, the exercises ahead, the time of day, activity prior to the warm-up and how you're feeling. You may need a long warm-up to get in the right frame of mind, or you might be raring to go.

Warming up before weight training

Prior to weight training, it's advisable to at least do the following:

- Perform some form of pulse raiser, like a jog, cycle or row. I favour rowing, as it exercises the arms as well as the legs.
- Perform some mobilisation around the joints to be exercised. This can either be very lightweight versions of the exercises to come, or movements similar to them. For example, if legs are about to be trained, bodyweight squats would be a good mobiliser. If the chest is about to be exercised, a few press-up movements in the air before a few slow press-ups themselves would be a good idea. Other useful mobilisers for the upper body include various swim-stroke arm movements.
- Perform light versions of the exercise to come, slowly building up the weight to the working weight. A good example would be 4–8 reps at 30% of working weight, 4–8 reps at 50% of working weight, 4–8 reps at 70% of working weight and 4–8 reps at 80% of working weight. Take a little rest between these, but not too much.
- Perform the session as outlined.
- When you start a new muscle group, ensure you perform step 3 above for that movement.

NB: With dips and pull-ups, use other similar exercises or machines to warm up the muscles.

Prior to leg training it's a good idea to 'switch on' the glutes, especially for ladies. To do this do glute bridges or clams.

Warming up before HIIT or LISS training

Perform a slow jog, cycle or row for two minutes depending on what your actual session will be. Then perform the following:

- Gently flick your toes out to the front for 10 reps.
- Gently bring your knees halfway up to your waist for 10 reps.
- Gently flick your heels halfway up to your rear for 10 reps.

Each should be done two or three times. Then raise the pulse again by running, cycling or rowing for 2–3 minutes, faster than originally performed.

After that, perform the following dynamic stretches:

- 5 slow squats to stretch the adductors and glutes (groin and backside).
- lunges on each leg to stretch the quadriceps (front of the thigh).
- 5 'Russian walks' on each leg (scraping the bottom of your shoe down an imaginary wall from as high as possible each time) to stretch the hamstrings (back of upper leg).

Leg swings can also be used, basically swinging the leg from the hip through its natural movement. Lastly run, cycle or row for a minute, then go into the HIIT or LISS session.

Cooling down after weights

After your resistance session, the most important thing is to start your recovery and, therefore, adaptations and progression. Consequently there are three things I see as important for your cool-down:

- Post-workout shake – see Chapter 4.
- A brief stretch of the muscles used in the session, to help reduce DOMS.

- A post-workout meal within an hour or so of drinking your shake.

To further aid recovery, use a foam roller or get a massage later in the day. A foam roller in front of the TV is a great option – it's something I do as often as possible, and I encourage all my clients to do the same.

Cooling down after HIIT or LISS

As above, the first thing to do (as long as you aren't going to be sick after a HIIT session!) is to have a post-workout shake. Following that, depending on where/when the session is taking place, all or none of the following should be performed:

- Reduce the amount of exercise but don't stop completely (or you could faint).
- Re-dress to avoid getting cold, unless at the gym and showering.
- Relax, by controlling your breathing and perhaps sitting or lying down.
- Stretch the muscles involved, but foam roll/massage again later.
- Eat within an hour of finishing.
- Trat any niggles or injuries (hopefully there'll be none).

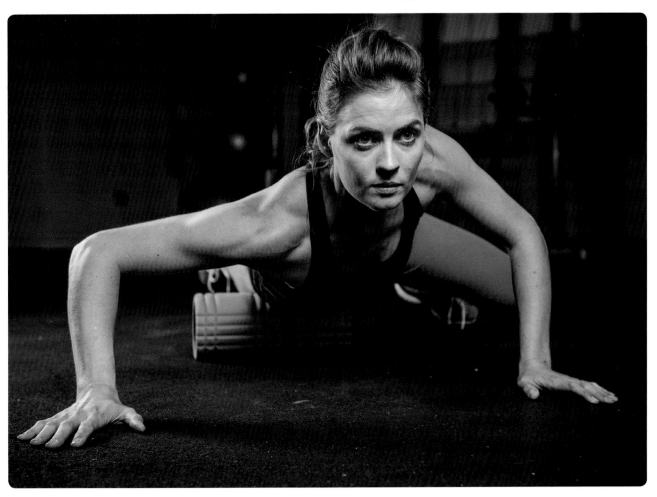

CHAPTER 4
NUTRITION

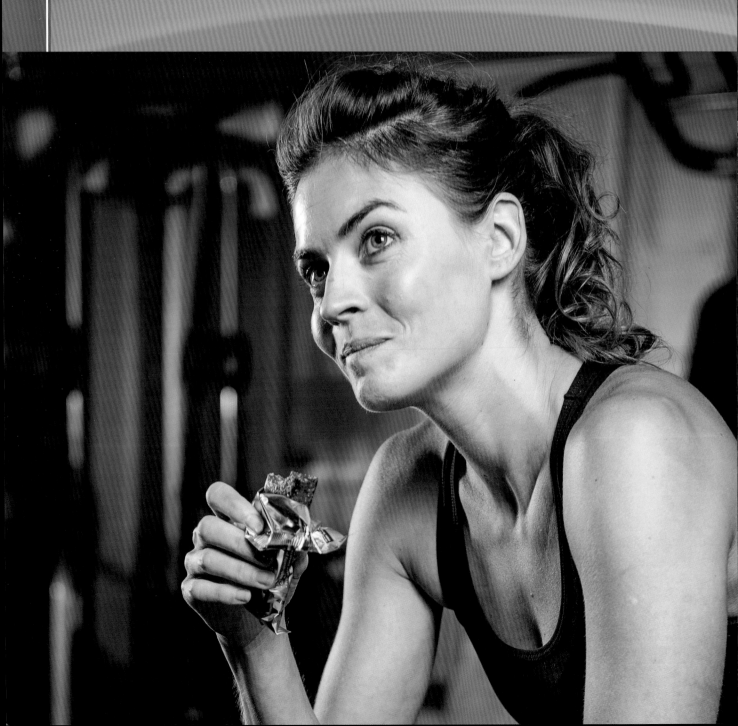

For 90% of the people who approach me for training, it's aesthetic results that they really want. I do get my fair share of people wanting to join the military, train for a marathon or triathlon, or increase their strength and conditioning for a sport, but even those with such ambitions often have an underlying goal of simply improving their physique. Regardless, the most fundamental thing to get right is nutrition. Not just what to eat and what not to eat, but when to eat.

As with everything in this book, I shall try to keep it simple. Therefore I'm going to advocate a basic calorific deficit (*ie* making sure you take in less calories than you need) while utilising a low-carb, moderate-fat, high-protein diet.

The simple reason for this is that I believe most of you will be eating more calories than you need, and probably eating a surplus of carbohydrate compared to what you really require. Eating carbohydrate prevents your body from using body fat as a fuel, so we want to lower it to coax the body into chipping away at the body fat that's hiding the figure or physique you really want to display. However, if we simply go to zero or very low carbohydrate you'll affect a whole host of hormones that require carbohydrate to function properly, not to mention possibly slow down the process of protein synthesis and muscle building. We'll therefore employ a low-carb diet at first, with one 'refeed' or 'cheat meal' a week, and then move on to the increasingly popular 'carb cycling' routine. Both these methods ensure you have higher carbohydrate on certain days (as your calorie needs increase from exercise) to pick up your body's natural normal balances, fuel your workouts and make you feel human. For example, on non-training days your calorie needs will be lower, hence so will your carbohydrate intake. Varying carb intake will hopefully make this 12-week process liveable and, more importantly, long-lasting. You may even be able to continue it beyond your 12-week programme.

Protein

The nutrients that your body needs in the largest quantities are called macronutrients, of which there are three: protein, fats and carbohydrates. Of these, I suspect that most of you aren't getting anywhere near enough of is protein – especially as the RDA (recommended dietary allowance) of 0.8g/kg is well under what research would indicate we really need. When training hard, we need to ensure protein synthesis is switched on and remains on so that we can build muscle, lower body fat and thus build a physique to be proud of. To do that we simply need to ensure you're eating enough protein. Research doesn't suggest any ill effects from eating too much protein, and as we're lowering carbs but still need you to hit your calorie requirements, we can make up the necessary calories using protein. Research suggests between 1.5–2.5g/kg of protein for strength/power athletes. However, I usually use 1.5g/lb of body weight, which is a standard across the industry when putting someone through a transformation. This is closer to 3.3g/kg. I'd therefore say a minimum of 2.5g/kg and up to 3.3g/kg of protein is needed for each of you.

So let's say that middle ground of 3g/kg would be a good starting point for the body compositional change nutritional plan for this programme, without hampering carb and fat intake, and, of course, while still staying in a calorie deficit.

To help you feel full, increase your protein synthesis, try to keep you anabolic (*ie* stop muscle breakdown) and feel like you're still eating a decent amount of food, we're going to up your protein intake and get you to eat vegetables with (almost) every meal.

It's not about a diet, it's about making sensible choices to support your training, lifestyle and aesthetic needs.

Timing is everything

You need to be very selective regarding *when* you eat. Try to put most of your daily carbs around training to fuel the session, utilise the carbs in the session and protect your muscle from breakdown. I'm not a fan of enforcing, saying you MUST do this or do that, as everyone is different and being overly dogmatic or restrictive can hinder compliance and make you 'fall off the wagon', so to speak. However, most of you doubtless skip breakfast or just have carbs (cereal or toast), so we need to get you eating protein at breakfast. It doesn't have to be just protein, although some people do find that a protein-only breakfast helps them keep carbohydrate lower over the whole day. A breakfast of eggs, steak or good quality beef burgers, or 'old-fashioned' fish like kippers, with a side of spinach, would be a great start to the day if you fall into that category. Having said that, research has shown that our insulin levels and body in general is more primed for carbohydrate in the morning, and

 Personal preference

Personal preference in food and diet is the number one thing that's overlooked when many trainers are designing a nutritional programme, yet it's the most important thing in ensuring long-term compliance and adherence.

that actually having a higher portion of carbs at breakfast (still with a good portion of protein) can actually help with getting leaner faster. Again, different strokes for different folks. I've tried both, myself and with clients, and found that both have worked with different people.

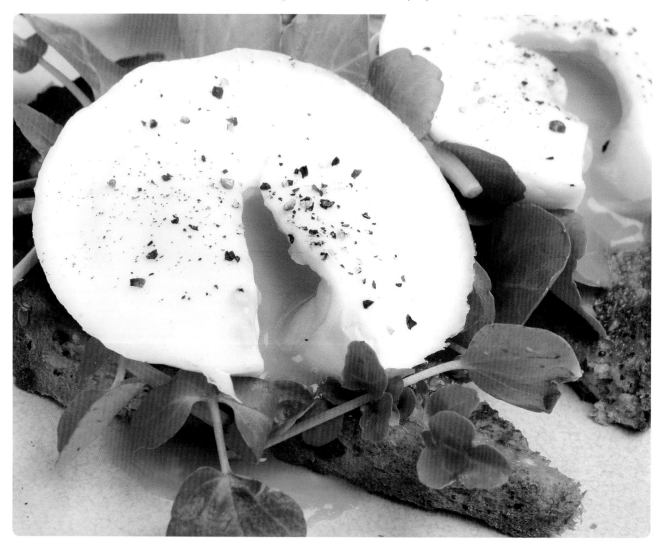

Eating to lose fat

Lowering your body fat is also down to nutrition. In fact, many go as far as to say that it's 70% down to nutrition and only 30% to exercise. A good nutrition plan firstly involves getting rid of the foods that are making you fat. Nope, they aren't necessarily those that contain fat, they're the crisps, chocolate, biscuits, cakes (all containing fat and carbs together) and alcohol that you know you shouldn't have, along with all the fruit you eat when you 'eat healthily' for a day or so. Fruits are a superb source of natural vitamins and minerals, but they are very high in sugar. They're also easy – apple, orange, banana – so think of them as 'fast food' and limit their intake to one piece in the morning and one piece straight after exercise or a couple of pieces spread through the day on your higher carb days as a natural source of sugars to refuel the body. Berries are a good substitute for fruit as they have a different ratio of sugars (sugars can be sucrose, fructose or glucose and don't all act in the same way), and are full of antioxidants to help your body rid itself of the free radicals your daily life, diet and training cause. However, that isn't an excuse to eat punnets of berries: your food intake needs to be varied and, remember, protein-rich.

Wherever possible, though, 'think greens': eat greens and non-starchy vegetables like spinach, broccoli and cauliflower, as they contain far more nutrients than a lot of fruits but far less carbohydrate. As we're limiting carbs, this will be a big help! They'll also fill you up.

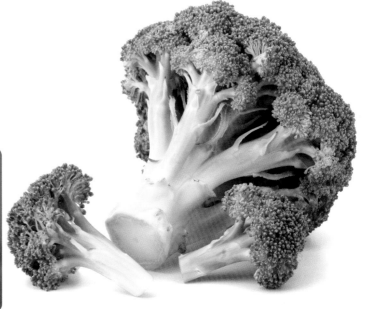

Fruit

Although high in carbohydrate (sugars), fruits are not bad! We need to make sure we hit our individual macronutrient needs of proteins, carbohydrates and fats, and within that you can eat your fair share of fruit up to your carbohydrate allowance for that day.

Fats

As well as choosing the right food, adequate protein and the right amount of carbs to ensure you lose body fat while keeping everything working correctly, we also need a good amount of the third macronutrient: fat.

Fats have acquired a really bad reputation, to the point where we try our best to avoid them. This is fundamentally wrong. They aren't to be avoided – in fact the right fats are actually good for you and far better than some carbs, *ie* highly sugary foods. The reason we've learnt to avoid them is that fats are 9 calories per gram, versus only 4 calories per gram for protein and carbohydrate. Therefore, the old thought process was to limit them and thereby lower calories. The problem with this is that the body needs good fats to function properly, not to mention to get the body to utilise fat as a fuel.

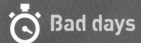

Bad days

A bad day of eating – eating well in excess of your calorie needs, especially if alcohol is involved – doesn't just cancel out one good day, it cancels around four good days.

For example, a simple rule is that if less than quarter of a person's bodyweight in pounds comes from good sources of dietary fat, it can have adverse effects on certain hormones, like testosterone. Testosterone is necessary for muscle growth, so really important for a transformation – not to mention male libido.

Changing the way you eat

During my time in the Marines, working as a Marine PTI undertaking any physically arduous course, I was fit, but not as lean as I am now. Obtaining the lean physique that I now have, with some added muscle since my Marine days, has allowed me to work professionally as a sports model. I managed to lower my body fat considerably by using a style of eating called 'carb cycling' – a process of changing the amount of carbohydrate you eat over a series of days, from no carbs to low/medium to high carbs.

The reason I was so specific, at the beginning of this programme, about committing 100% to this process, is that carb cycling – like the training itself – can be tough. Furthermore, I don't see it as a diet: it's a way of life. If you stick to the ideas behind the way to eat set out below, for the length of your transformation, you'll lower your body fat and obtain the physique you want by combining it with a correctly administered exercise and training regime. Once you're finished, you can step away from carb cycling at any point – for example when you're on holiday, at Christmas, when you want to take a few weeks' rest or for whatever other reason you decide. Then you can come back to it and utilise it to again reach your goals. To emphasise, this can become a way of life around your lifestyle, work, training and social life, to help you keep the figure or physique you want while still enjoying life.

Eat right to look good

As you'll have gathered by now, the secret to obtaining a great physique isn't just in the training. After all, even if you trained for an hour every day, that's still only seven of the 168 hours in a week, which is 4.2%. In fact you'll probably be doing around four or five hours. Even at the end of this programme you'll be doing at most three to four 15–20 minute morning LISS (low intensity steady state) cardiovascular sessions and five to six training sessions of 45–60 minutes per week. That equates to a maximum of 7 hours 20 minutes – still under 5% of your available time.

So, what's important then? Well, like I said previously, *everything else* – everything you do in those 23 other hours per day, or those other 160 hours per week that you're not training, from sleeping, to working, to resting, to ... yes, eating. Arguably THE most important aspect of changing your body's composition is what you eat, and when you eat it.

Don't take this the wrong way, but most of you reading this will be eating terribly. Your food choices will be based around fast food, supermarket lunches and supermarket deals. The majority of you will be eating too much carbohydrate and too little protein and will consider fat bad, preferring sugary treats to keep you going through the day. Sound familiar? No? I beg to differ. The following is an example of a regular person's day, and I bet it sounds familiar:

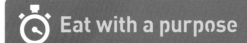

Eat with a purpose

Everything that passes your lips should have a nutritional value, not just look and taste good.

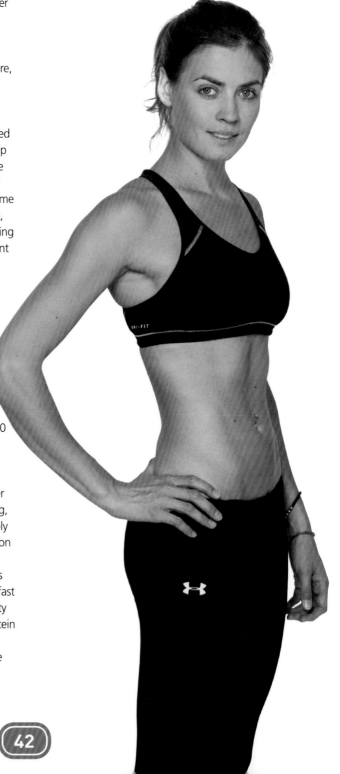

Typical 'regular' diet

Breakfast

Bowl of cereal 50g carbs
Milk 12g carbs
Banana 24g carbs
Tea with milk and one teaspoon of sugar 5g carbs
Total 91g carbohydrate

Mid-morning break

Tea with milk and one teaspoon of sugar 5g carbs
A couple of biscuits @ 9g/biscuit 18g carbs
Total 23g carbohydrate

Lunch

Takeaway sandwich 37g carbs
Medium apple 20g carbs
Medium orange 15g carbs
Fruit juice drink 26g carbs
Muesli bar 19g carbs
Total 117g carbohydrate

Afternoon snack

Tea with milk and one teaspoon of sugar 5g carbs
Doughnut 26g carbs
Total 31g carbohydrate

Dinner

Salad 0g carbs
Steak 0g carbs
Pasta 30g carbs
Bread roll 29g carbs
Couple of glasses of wine @ 4g/glass 8g carbs
Ice cream bar 21g carbs
Total 88g carbohydrate

TV snack

Chocolate bar 34g carbs

Day total = 384g carbohydrate

Example low carb

Breakfast

3 large eggs 2g carbs
Bacon 0g carbs
Green tea 0g carbs
Total 2g carbohydrate

Mid-morning

Water 0g carbs
Coffee with milk 3g carbs
10–15 almonds @ 0.24g/nut 3g carbs
Total 6g carbohydrate

Lunch

Salad (2 cups) with assorted vegetables (including tomatoes/carrot/peppers) 6g carbs
Chicken breast 0g carbs
Cheese (3oz) 1g carbs
Water 0g carbs
Total 7g carbohydrate

Snack

Green tea 0g carbs
Celery/carrot sticks (3 of each) 3g carbs
Peanut butter (100%) 2.9g carbs
Total 6g carbohydrate

Dinner

Half a roasted chicken 0g carbs
Broccoli (2 cups) 7g carbs
Mixed salad (4 cups) 2g carbs
Peanut butter (100%) and olive oil satay sauce 2.9g carbs
Water 0g carbs
Total 12g carbohydrate

TV snack

Blueberries half a cup 10g carbs

Day total = 43g carbohydrate

⏱ Count your carbs

NB. I am not saying carbohydrate is bad. I am not advocating no-carb diets. What I am saying is that in the world we live in, we rely on them too much. They are easy and cheap and thus we over-eat them. Would that be a problem if we weren't trying to obtain a better figure/physique? Perhaps not. But we are. However, we still need carbs for the reasons mentioned previously, so the message is to be aware, not cut out!

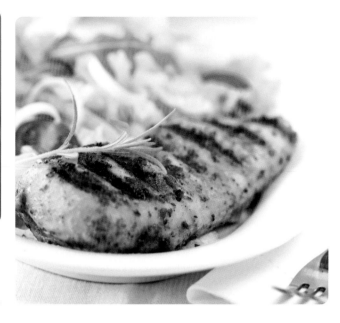

Now remember, if your body has carbohydrate it won't use body fat for fuel. If it has more carbohydrate than it needs (if you're in a daily calorific surplus) then it'll store the excess carbohydrate as fat. It doesn't matter if the excess is fruit (yes, healthy fruit!), if it's more than your body needs you'll put on body fat. So, that 384g of carbs from the list on the previous page, that equates to 1,536 calories. That's without including any of the protein or fats from the day's diet. You can see how easy it is to take in too many calories and, in particular, too much carbohydrate.

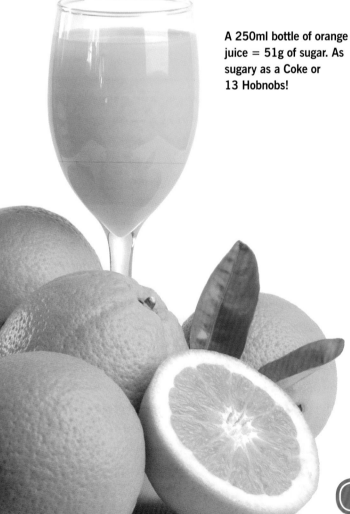

A 250ml bottle of orange juice = 51g of sugar. As sugary as a Coke or 13 Hobnobs!

Yes, these two 'days' represent two completely opposite ends of the scale, and I'm not suggesting that everyone needs to adopt the latter at all. Each person is different and requires a different number of calories and carbohydrates. However, my point is that the first example isn't actually that bad (there's no real junk food or fast food), yet the carbohydrates have ramped up very quickly. (So imagine the impact of a *bad* day of crisps, chocolate, fast-food burger and chips, and a cake or bun with coffee, etc...) By contrast, the second 'day' shows that a few sensible options can make a real difference.

Therefore, by initially getting you to choose 'better' food sources, not only will you start to see changes (hopefully), but you'll also feel a whole lot better and have more energy, and therefore the training part becomes a fair bit easier.

Guidelines

People often get too bound up in the complicated nutrition messages from various sources, when, to put it simply, if you're over 20% body fat the key is to simply make the changes opposite:

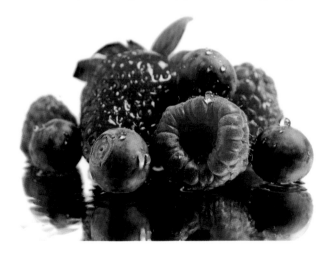

The seven rules to lower your body fat during the first two weeks

1 Only eat high quality food choices – real, natural, foods rather than refined foods. If it hasn't grown from the ground or in a tree, lived, swam or run and had a face, don't eat it.

2 Ensure you're in a calorie deficit necessary to lose fat. To do this, eat 5–20% less than your requirements from the workings below.

3 Ensure you eat enough protein to maintain the lean muscle mass you have. A minimum of 2.5g/kg of bodyweight according to research, though I recommend around 3g/kg is optimal, especially for males undertaking a training programme like the one laid out in this book.

4 Ensure 25–30% of your daily calorie intake is from fats – good quality 'good fats' from oily fish, avocado, meat, butter and nuts.

5 The rest of your calories are made up of carbohydrate, the amount of which is calculated from the remainder after calculating your protein and fat needs. Choose real foods like sweet potatoes, basmati rice and oats for carbs.

6 Eat the number of meals a day that suits your lifestyle and working day, but ensure a good distribution of the food and macronutrients that allows you to most consistently stick with this new way of eating and maximise your training. Eating 20g of protein every three hours has been shown to keep protein synthesis and stop catabolism. This can be a good base for you meals.

7 Have a 'cheat' meal (I don't like the term, but hey, it paints a picture) twice a month or once a week, to ensure you can keep to the plan long-term. Once you've finished that meal and left the table, that's it. Back to good eating for the week.

It gets more complicated as body fat lowers, but until then just make a start. Follow these seven guidelines, be as consistent and patient as possible, train hard and start to see changes.

Cheat meals or refeeds while following the seven rules

To reiterate, you need to lower carbohydrate intake to ensure body fat is lowered, but you need high carbohydrate intake to reset hormonal balance. Hence 'refeed' (or 'cheat') days/meals. People often speak about high carb days or meals cranking up metabolism, but this theory isn't actually very research-supported. If it is the case, it's very minor. However, a high-carb day/meal does reset hormonal balance, refuel glycogen and, most importantly for many, improve mood!

It's important to not go over the calorie intake needed for the day when you refeed or 'cheat'. It's OK to go over the 5–20% defect you've calculated, but it's important not to go over the original starting figure required for maintenance. (See workings in the next column.)

Number of refeed days needed, dependent on body fat

2 per month if over 15–20%.
1 per week under 15%.
2 per week under 10%.

Linear diet

The seven guidelines listed in the previous column are for a basic linear diet, or at least the start of one. What most people would do is to continue to cut calories (because their weight drops as they lose body fat, so their calorie needs become less (as per calculations shown below), so they just continue cutting calories until they reach their goal. At least, that's the plan.

This unfortunately rarely works long-term. It's not just a huge struggle, as the body constantly tries to reach homeostasis and work with what it's given; it also often leads to huge weight rebound when the dieter returns to more 'normal' eating/calorie levels. They literally balloon, often bigger than where they started. How many times have we seen this in celebrity magazines?

The human body is highly adaptive and craves regularity/homeostasis. It therefore adapts to any calorie deficit. This means you either have to increase the amount of exercise (think of those women you see at the gym doing two hours of cross-trainer every day) or lower the calories again, and again. Yet the body will still fight to restore homeostasis. In the end the effect is that the longer someone diets like this, the harder it becomes to continue lowering body fat and getting the oh-so-desired results.

Without getting too scientific, this is because of a very important hormone called leptin, which is produced less and less during dieting and restricted calorie intake. Simply put, reduced leptin levels increase hunger and cravings while slowing the metabolic rate (meaning your body needs less calories to function) and reducing energy expenditure. You literally crave more, but need less, all because of consistent dieting. Not only is this enough to drive someone crazy, but it explains why no one can keep this going sanely, and why people 'bounce back'.

To make matters worse, leptin is what we call a 'master control hormone'. This means its levels (high or low) have an effect on other hormones. Yes, you've guessed it, during long periods of calorie deficit low leptin levels affect the levels of testosterone, growth hormone, IGF-1 and thyroid. All the men reading this will now be devastated, knowing that low testosterone and GH can negatively impact not just their muscle growing, but their sex lives! Men, I've won you over already, right?

However, you women will probably be thinking, 'I can live with low testosterone and GH levels.' But what if I told you low GH levels mean you'll show signs of ageing quicker – more wrinkles, thin skin, age spots, lack of 'muscle tone', more fat? I had you with more wrinkles on the face, didn't I? With me again? Good.

So we all agree that continual cutting of calories to try and obtain the perfect figure or physique isn't worth it if it means we'll either bounce back to twice the size, go nuts from food cravings or age quicker (ladies) or have no sex drive (guys)? Great. So how do we do it, then?

Carb cycling

As I mentioned at the beginning of this chapter, carb cycling is the answer. Whereas basic calorific deficit works for lowering body fat at the higher end, the lower your body fat becomes (under 15–20%), the more difficult things become. As I say about anything difficult, whether it's obtaining a green beret, a medical degree or winning a gold medal, if it was easy everyone would achieve it. If everyone achieved it, it would cease to be special and no one would want it anymore.

So embrace the difficulty, use it to spur you on. That way, when you succeed the success is so much sweeter. However, with less percentage body fat to lose you have less leeway for mistakes and more danger of breaking down muscle.

Men, I know you won't want to lose muscle: what's the point of having sub 10% body fat if you look like you've been stranded on a desert island for six months?

Women, you'll be thinking 'I don't mind losing some muscle.' Well you should. If you're letting your body break down muscle, it's not breaking down fat, and you want it to do that. Second, muscle is your metabolic tissue: it uses the calories you put in. The more (muscle) you have, the more you need to eat. Wouldn't it be nicer

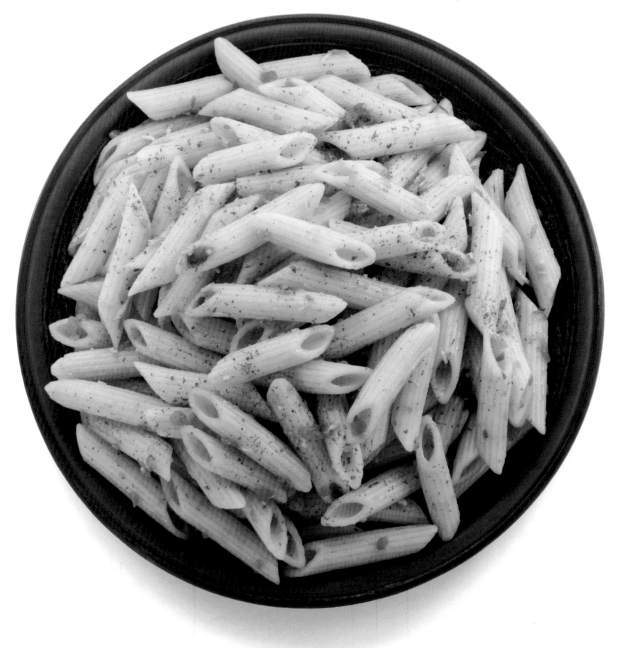

to be able to enjoy decent meals (and cheat meals) because you have more metabolic muscle tissue on your body?

Letting your body break down muscle to fuel it, effectively sabotaging your metabolism with improper dieting methods, is what we absolutely need to avoid. It's what anorexic people do, and it is very difficult to come back from.

Simply put, we want to cause the opposite effects to the body's systems while still continuing to reduce body fat, and we do that by periodic calorie surpluses. We give the body excess calories occasionally, thus having the exact opposite effects of chronic caloric restriction. By giving the human body a one-day 'refeed' (I hate the term, it makes us sound like cattle, but it's essentially what we're doing), it can offset the metabolic downshift that occurs with dieting – that desire of the body to reach homeostasis. Not only that, the excess calories re-boost leptin, and thus testosterone, growth hormone and thyroid to normal pre-diet levels. Exactly what we need to occur. Genius? Not really. It's simple, but how many people do you know who do this?

I discovered carb cycling after I left the Marines and decided to become a personal trainer and professional sports model. I use carb cycling myself and with my clients. It allows you to trim body fat while maintaining all of your hard-earned and (ladies) much-needed muscle. Furthermore, it prevents the metabolic and hormonal drawbacks of more extreme yet more mainstream dieting.

If you've been dieting for a while and have simply hit a plateau, you may find that introducing carb cycling will re-sensitise your body to fat-burning, and you'll literally see a huge improvement after a few weeks and lose that last layer of fat that's been refusing to budge.

Body fat 15% and over – refeed twice a month

If you still have what you consider to be a large amount of body fat to lose, it's best to ensure that the majority of the time you continue in a calorie deficit, just as you would have been from my initial seven points. Therefore, for all but two days a month eat your base fat-loss diet as shown in the workings below: 30% calories from good fats, 2.5–3g/kg protein and the rest from carbohydrate. Eat this way on both training and non-training days.

Then, twice a month, spike calories to maintenance levels (original figure below before 5–20% cut for fat loss). Keep fats the same as the original calculation, keep protein the same, and increase carbs to make up the excess, meaning all calorie increase is from carbohydrate. This increased amount of carbs in turn increases leptin levels. Carbs do this more so than good fats or protein, which is why excess calories should be mostly carbohydrate-based. The only other rule is that these 'high carb days' occur on the same day as your most intense training sessions. For most, this is a leg session, an interval (HIIT) day or an all-over body day containing big compound movements.

Body fat under 15% – refeed once a week

Keep things as above. Most days you eat your calorific deficit and keep your proteins and fats as stated, making the rest of you calories from carbs. However, now, once a week, you have a higher day (on your leg or interval training days) and raise calories up to the non 5–20% cut, the increase coming mostly from carbohydrate. Sounds complicated, but it isn't. See the example below.

Body fat 10% or under – refeed twice a week

With body fat under 10% you can afford to have two high days a week. It's still the same as the last two examples, just more frequent. Again, time the higher days to coincide with your most intense training days, like legs or intervals.

But, but, but...

Although I'm advising the carb cycle form outlined above, it isn't the only way it's done. There are many different ways to carb cycle. I actually try different versions with different clients at different times. Some work for certain people, some work for others, in terms of their body composition and their lifestyle/compliance. Other examples include high day once a week (highest calories on leg day), no-carb days on rest days (carbs only from cruciferous veg) and low-carb days on all other training days (calories 20% less than maintenance calories). This works well, but involves more variation and I believe will be more confusing in this book. However, it's an option if you want it.

Variation is key

People say consistency is key, and I broadly agree, but I also think that if you consistently do something that just isn't working you'll just stay the same. So I'm a big believer in variation – you need to vary things to get results: we know this is true in the gym – up the weights, shorten the rest time, anything to make it harder than before to force change. Hence variation is key. Having said that, one article I read while researching for this book said of carb cycling that 'it doesn't seem to matter how you do it, the main thing is, carb cycling works'. And I guess for me, that's the take-home message.

Conclusion

There is no 'one size fits all' to fat loss/body composition. You need to work out your calorie needs, your protein needs, your fat needs, and then vary your carb needs according to where you are percentage body-fat-wise. If that sounds like too much hassle, then ask yourself if this book and programme is really for you. There are no quick fixes here... Again (repeat after me), if it was easy everyone would do it...

Try things, test them, assess, adjust, test, readjust etc. Find what works for you, your lifestyle, your body, your work. Just don't give up, and if you don't I (almost!) guarantee that this eating style, coupled with the training programme, will see you looking the part in your shorts or bikini on your next holiday.

Time for the maths

The following examples show how I think you can best calculate your calorie needs. There are other methods, but from the many methods I've seen and tried with my clients I think this is the quickest and simplest, yet still the most accurate of them all. It's loosely based on a method used by Joseph Agu, a performance nutritionist at the English Institute of Sport who works with British Athletics. I've found his method great for designing diets for sportsmen and those wanting strength and conditioning, but have tweaked it for my fat-loss clients.

The basics

To keep matters simple we need to work out two things to estimate your calorie needs:

1. BMR – the energy needed to sustain you at rested state each day.
2. TEA/TEF – the energy needed for all physical activity, both voluntary (exercise) and involuntary (shivering, fidgeting etc); and the thermic effects of the macronutrients during digestion, *ie* the energy needed to digest foods eaten.

To obtain a good BMR value for calculating a body transformation diet, multiply your weight in kilos by 22. (However, if you're an active male, looking at building muscle, use 24.2 instead.)

Once you have the BMR, you then multiply that value by an assigned activity factor from the list below that takes into account TEA and TEF. For most of you following this programme, your activity factor will be 1.55 (three to five training days per week). This will provide a value of calories that you need in order to maintain weight (maintenance calories) at that level of activity.

Activity factors

Sedentary	BMR x 1.2
Little/no exercise and an inactive desk job	
Light activity	BMR x 1.375
Play a sport or perform light exercise 1–3 days per week	
Moderate activity	BMR x 1.55
Moderate exercise 3–5 days per week	
High activity	BMR x 1.725
Hard exercise 6–7 days per week	
Excess activity	BMR x 1.9
Hard daily exercise and physical job or twice-a-day training	

To ensure a calorific deficit, this must be reduced by 5–20%. Some people believe reducing by 5% each week every couple of weeks to reach 20% is better than dropping straight to 20%. I believe this is up to the individual. If you're a strong-minded, strong-willed person, going straight to 20% is probably fine. If you're not, then start with just a 5% drop and then drop a further 5% each week or two until you're at 20%.

Examples

Let's take a 100kg man and a 60kg woman – probably pretty average for our 'overweight' individuals signing up to transform their body composition with this book.

I say 'overweight' in inverted commas, as they aren't overweight really, just 'over-fat' and 'under-muscled'. They may well weigh more at the end of the process, as muscle weighs more than fat. But we don't care about weight. We care about body composition.

SEE EXAMPLES OPPOSITE

Confused? You shouldn't be. This is just simple maths. Read it again and take it slow. The things you need to know are:

Carbs are 4 calories per gram
Protein is 4 calories per gram
Fats are 9 calories per gram

Your calculation for calorie needs will be:
22kcal/kg for BMR.
× 1.55 activity level for calorie requirements.
– 20% decrease for maintenance calories for fat loss.

You simply work out your macronutrient amounts from there.
30% fats.
2.5–3g/kg protein (aim for 3g if you can).
The rest comes from carbs.

As I've said throughout, there is no one size fits all. If, after a few weeks of following this, you really can't see any changes, then tweak your calorie deficit value. Take it down by 5% and work out your carbs again. Give this another couple of weeks and see what happens. Eventually you'll find what works for you. Just stick at it and be honest with yourself. If you're sneaking biscuits at work and having glasses of wine in the evening, it definitely won't work!

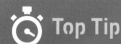 Top Tip

Get the free MyFitnessPal app on your smartphone. Use it to log everything you eat. It has a barcode scanner, or you can search other people's entries. It has a huge, huge database. You can adjust portion sizes for others weights/sizes. It's THE tool to use to enable you to see how many carbs one apple or one sweet potato has really given you.

100kg male

Calorie needs (22cal per kg to get BMR):
22 x 100kg = 2,200kcal per day
× Activity factor = 1.55 (moderately active)
2,200 × 1.55 = 3,410kcal
− Reduce by 20% to create calorific deficit:
3,410 ÷ 100 × 80 =   **2,728kcal**

Calorie needs are made up of Fats, Protein and Carbohydrates:

Fats (30% of daily calories are obtained from fats) so:
2,728 ÷ 100 × 30 =   **818kcal**
Fats are 9 calories per gram, so
818 ÷ 9 = 90.9g of good fats per day.

Protein (3g per kg), so
3 × 100 = 300g of protein per day
Remember, minimum protein is 2.5g/kg,
so total could be 250g if necessary.
Protein is 4 calories per gram, so
4 x 300g =   **1,200kcal**

Carbohydrate: so far we have −
90.9g of fat   818kcal
300g of protein   1,200kcal
                       2,018kcal
Remaining calorie needs to be obtained from carbs:
2,728 − 2,018 =   **710kcal**
Carbohydrates are 4 calories per gram, so
710 ÷ 4 = 178g of carbs per day

DAILY TOTAL	Fat	90.9g	818kcal
	Protein	300g	1,200kcal
	Carbohydrates	178g	710kcal
			2,728kcal

Don't forget the cheat meal/refeed meal when it comes around.
Calorie needs are now increased to original non-deficit value:
3,410kcal per day (22cal/kg × 100kg × 1.55 activity level).

Fat stays the same @ 90.9g =   818kcal
Protein stays the same @ 300g =   1,200kcal
                                     2,018kcal

So carbohydrates increase to:
3,410kcal − 2,018kcal =   **1,392kcal**
1,392 ÷ 4 =   **348g carbs**

60kg female

Calorie needs (22cal/kg (to get BMR):
22 x 60kg = 1,320kcal per day
× Activity factor = 1.55 (moderately active)
1,320 × 1.55 = 2,046kcal
− Reduce by 20% to create calorific deficit:
2,046 ÷ 100 × 80 =   **1,637kcal**

Calorie needs are made up of Fats, Protein and Carbohydrates:

Fats (30% of daily calories are obtained from fats) so:
1,637 ÷ 100 × 30 =   **491kcal**
Fats are 9 calories per gram, so
491 ÷ 9 = 54.5g of good fats per day.

Protein (3g per kg), so
3 × 60 = 180g of protein per day
Remember, minimum protein is 2.5g/kg,
so total could be 150g if necessary.
Protein is 4 calories per gram, so
4 x 180g =   **720kcal**

Carbohydrate: so far we have
54.5g of fat   491kcal
180g of protein   720kcal
                       1,211kcal
Remaining calorie needs to be obtained from carbs:
1,637 − 1,211 =   **426kcal**
Carbohydrates are 4 calories per gram, so
426 ÷ 4 = 106.5g of carbs per day

DAILY TOTAL	Fat	54.5g	491kcal
	Protein	180g	720kcal
	Carbohydrates	106.5g	426kcal
			1,637kcal

Don't forget the cheat meal/refeed meal when it comes around.
Calorie needs are now increased to original non-deficit value:
2,046kcal per day (22cal/kg x 60kg x 1.55 activity level).

Fat stays the same @ 54.5 g =   491kcal
Protein stays the same @ 180g =   720kcal
                                     1,211kcal

So carbohydrates increase to:
2,046kcal − 1,211kcal =   **835kcal**
835 ÷ 4 =   **209g**

Alternative methods

For some people the idea of counting calories/carbs puts them off. They can't even think about doing it, whether for personal or work reasons, and therefore won't progress with a transformation. Although I can empathise with this way of thinking, try to get over it – use MyFitnessPal and give it a go: the results will come, and you may surprise yourself.

However, for those of you who simply can't or won't, there is an alternative that's not as complicated, eliminates the counting and focuses on the big picture. It may not be as reliable, but it'll allow you to carb cycle effectively and thus reap the anabolic benefits of carbohydrates while maintaining insulin sensitivity and (hopefully) keeping fat gain at bay. Other good reasons to adopt the alternative we're going to set out below are:

1 It's the way I personally got into carb cycling.
2 Counting calories and macros is a stress that some people can't live with. As I've said, what we're trying to achieve here is a lifestyle, not a diet, so it needs to be as easy as possible and complimentary to your life, in order to ensure compliance.

3 Certain people become unhealthily obsessed with counting macros and calories, and this can often lead to eating disorders or an unhealthy addiction to food/fitness, which impacts on relationships and other areas of life.
4 As I've explained, the types of food you *should* eat are those that have grown, lived, swam, moved or once had a face. The problem is, their values can still vary massively dependent on a number of factors, from how the animal was reared and what it was fed on, to what type of soil the vegetable was grown in, what pesticides were used and whether it's a GM product or organic etc. Hence their nutrient values will vary hugely, even before we start weighing them.
5 The cut of meat similarly means that its fat/protein content can vary significantly. As shown already, fat is 9kcal/g whereas protein is 4kcal/g, so a fatty piece of steak compared to a lean piece of the same size will vary considerably.
6 Nutritional labels for produced foods are usually based on average samples taken, which means you can't be 100%

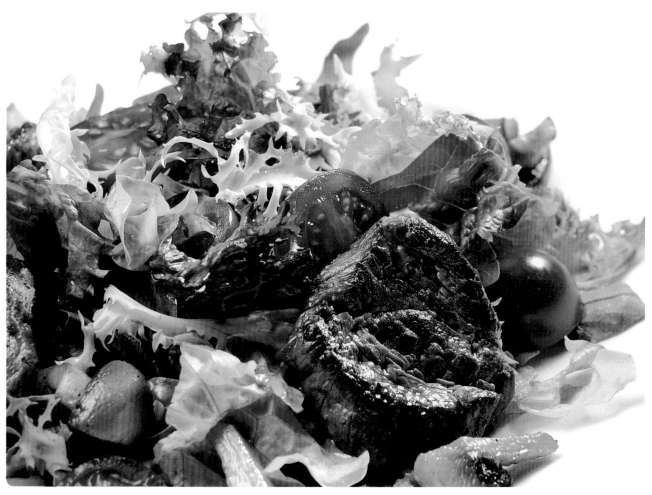

exact if you're counting macros – meaning you may be wasting your time trying to be that precise.

7 Energy expenditure calculations like those I've shown aren't 100% accurate: the variables considered, such as weight, all vary hugely from person to person. This is yet another reason why there can never be a 'one size fits all' solution: everyone is different, and invariably everyone's calculations need tweaking to make them as close to 'perfect' as possible.

8 Finally, it's worth considering the thermal effect of feeding (TEF) – whatever you eat, there's a thermal effect, *ie* the amount of energy that's used to digest the food. The accepted estimate is that 10% of energy consumed is used in digestion and assimilation of that food. However, this is seriously affected by factors such as food type (fats, protein, carbs), amount and type of fibre, type and quality of food, your individual insulin-sensitivity, your genetics and your lifestyle up to this point.

All this means that it's difficult to assign specific macronutrient and calorific amounts needed for the body, as it's really hard to determine an accurate baseline of what the body needs in order to operate. In reality the calculations given are therefore only an educated guess.

I can hear you now: 'So why spend loads of time and effort weighing, counting, and tracking food when the numbers probably aren't accurate'? Again, science has given us the calculations and results have shown that some people can live by their macros and use them to obtain great physiques. Often the numbers need fiddling, since, as I've said, there's no 'one size fits all' norm, but in general the scheme I've given is a great start. Still, some people find it far more liveable to just count carbs, eat protein every three hours and ensure they carb cycle.

If you'd prefer to count your macros, just follow the outline and example given and skip this section. However, if, like some of my clients, you're often away on business, so literally can't count your macros, then perhaps the following version is for you.

It's your choice.

'Carb only counting' carb cycling

You'll have three general days:

1. No-carb days – less than 50g carbs in a day.
2. Low-carb days – from 50–150g in a day.
3. High-carb days – from 250–500g in a day.

Simply put, you use the same basic guidelines as those given with the calorie counting and awareness of grams of carbs, fats and proteins, but instead of weighing everything you simply self-regulate and eat the amount it takes for you to feel satiated. Obviously, stick primarily to proteins and vegetables to make you feel full, except on high-carb days, when it's imperative to 'refuel' with carbohydrates.

This style of carb cycling is designed to avoid micromanaging,

but requires you to be sensible and (yes, here it comes again) 'know thyself'. So, don't overindulge, especially on the fats and the carbs – you probably need less food than you think. Having said that, don't starve yourself either. You can't afford to cut too many calories (around 500kcal) from your actual maintenance needs or you won't get the right results.

High days
Your high days should coincide with your most intense or highest-priority training days. For most that would be a leg or HIIT day.

Medium days
A medium day is a training day but not the most intense session (not usually legs or HIIT).

Low days
Low days are either a non-training day or just non-resistance training (sports practice, pleasure exercise, bodyweight circuits, remedial/recovery work, etc).

High carb frequency
As above, twice a month if over 15–20%, once a week under 15%, twice a week under 10%.

An example week
A typical week could look like this for someone with under 10% body fat:

Monday	Leg session, high day.
Tuesday	Upper body session, medium day.
Wednesday	No training, low day.
Thursday	HIIT session, high day.
Friday	Upper body session, medium day.
Saturday	No training, low day.
Sunday	No training, low day.

Or like this for someone with under 15% body fat:

Monday	Leg session, medium day.
Tuesday	Upper body session, medium day.
Wednesday	No training, low day.
Thursday	HIIT session, high day.
Friday	Upper body session, medium day.
Saturday	No training, low day.
Sunday	No training, low day.

As I hope I've drummed into you by now, there's no 'one size fits all', no perfect plan. This style of eating does work, but it's up to you to find the best way to utilise it. After two weeks, check your measurements, and if you think you're putting on too much fat reduce your portion sizes; or if you're doing two high-carb days a week, reduce this to one. It's all about working out what's best for your body.

Other factors

Some foods cause very common food intolerances, so if you're not making progress or are experiencing gastric problems, eliminating wheat, dairy, eggs or nuts for a time can be beneficial. However, do so one food at a time – otherwise you won't know which is the problem. Before you can positively point the finger of blame it's also important to give each food a decent time off (4–12 weeks) and then introduce it to see if the problems return.

Helpful portion sizes

■ Protein servings are one chicken breast, one tin of tuna: around 120–170g (that's the complete weight of the food, not the weight of protein they contain; protein content will be 20–30g max).
■ Vegetables are one cup.
■ Fruit is half a cup or one piece.
■ Fats are either the size of a golf ball (for nut butters, avocado), a tablespoon (for oils), or 15 nuts.
■ Carbs should be half a cup pre-cooked (oatmeal, brown rice) or one medium sweet potato.

Weight gain – hard gainers

There'll be some of you reading this who're thinking: 'This is all great, but my problem isn't that I need to cut body fat to reach the figure/physique I want, it's that I need to add some shape and muscle to my body.'

If that's you, don't worry, we're going to give you some guidelines here. Unlike the people who'll be carb cycling with a calorific deficit on one of the two plans given, you simply need to put surplus calories in, so that you can add some bodyweight – preferably muscle – and obtain the physique you want.

This isn't actually that complicated. You will have two days to worry about:

■ Training days.
■ Rest days.

You need around 24.2cal/kg of bodyweight multiplied by activity factor on training days and rest days. Protein-wise you need to have (as above) 2.5–3g/kg of bodyweight; 2.5 would be acceptable on rest days, but on training days try to get up to 3g using your protein shakes. Fat-wise, you need to be getting 30% of your calories from good fats. Carbs will make up the rest of your calories on both days.

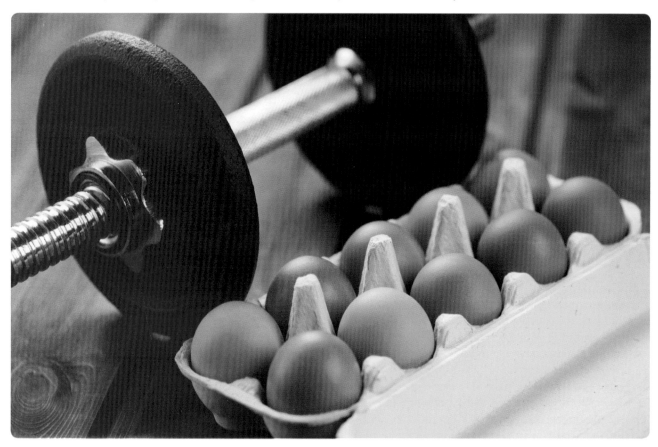

As an example we'll take a 70kg male:

Calorie needs (24.2 calories per kg)
24.2 × 70kg = 1,694kcal per day.
× Activity factor = 1.55 (moderately active)
1,694 × 1.55 =   **2,626kcal**
OR
× Activity factor = 1.725 if training very hard/extra session or find it very hard to add size
1,694 × 1.725 = 2,922kcal

Using first value (1.55):

Fats (30% of daily calories are obtained from fats) so:
2,626 ÷ 100 × 30 =   **788kcal**
Fats are 9 calories per gram, so
788 ÷ 9 = 87.5g of good fats per day.

Protein (3g per kg), so
3 x 70 = 210g of protein
Protein is 4 calories per gram, so
4 x 210g =   **840kcal**

Carbohydrate: so far we have –
87.5g of fat   788kcal
210g of protein   840kcal
               1628kcal
Daily calorie intake from carbs therefore
2,626 – 1628 =   **998kcal**
Carbohydrates are 4 calories per gram, so
998 ÷ 4 = 250g of carbs per day

DAILY TOTAL			
	Fat	87.5g	788kcal
	Protein	210g	840kcal
	Carbohydrates	250g	998kcal
			2,626kcal

That may seem complicated, but it isn't. Take a break, get a cup of (green) tea and read through the entire chapter again. Remember, carbs and proteins are 4cal per gram and fats are 9cal per gram. All you're doing then is multiplying your bodyweight in kg by some specific numbers I've given you. Simple!

If you find you put on too much weight doing this, then you can always go to the carb cycling plan to cut some body fat, but still utilise the resistance training and varying carb amounts to ensure some muscle growth.

The Non-Compliers

I know some of you out there will have got this far and be thinking: 'I can't do this' or 'This isn't for me'. There will be two reasons:

1. You don't want it enough. Until you do, I can't help you.
2. You just can't stand the thought of doing without your latte, or chocolate bar or smoothie etc.

If the latter is you, then you might find the following will allow you to carry on trying to get the figure/physique you want, while still having a little of what you like.

Still calculate your calorie deficit and protein, fat and carb requirements as already given. You then take off 250-400kcals from that figure. For example your calorie deficit requirements are 2,000kcal, so let's say you take off 300kcal, you have 1,700kcal. Eat 'perfectly' (as best you can) for your 1,700kcal – correct amounts of protein, fats and carbs throughout the day to make up that 1,700kcal. Then, your excess can be something you can't live without: more fruit, a smoothie, ice cream, chocolate etc. (I'd still avoid alcohol due to the negative effects on muscle building). Just ensure you stay within calories. If you do that, you can still get good results without completely sacrificing the things you love in life. Again, compliance is most important and if this helps you comply, then it's a better system for you.

Conclusion

On the first read-through this chapter will probably feel way too complicated, but it really isn't. So read it again, and remember that two of the things I say towards the beginning are:

1. That lowering your body fat is 70% down to nutrition and 30% down to exercise, so is it any real surprise that the chapter needs to be so detailed? Not really.
2. That it's going to challenge you, and that some of you will find it hard to stick at it. But the things we really want in life are hard to attain, which is why we want them.

Now you know what needs to be done. Are you ready to put in the effort?

CHAPTER 5
SUPPLEMENTS

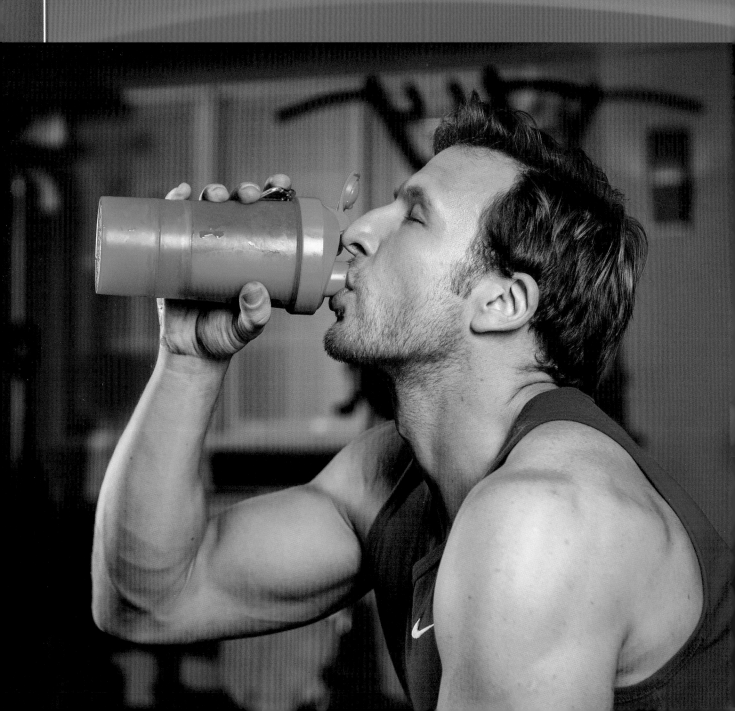

First things first. A supplement is a *supplement* – it isn't critical, it doesn't destroy the whole process if you don't want to take it or can't afford it. Yes, it can aid progress and perhaps give you a better result, but I'd always place good-quality wholesome food above supplements. So remember, supplements supplement your diet, they don't replace it.

Despite what I've just said, supplements can help a lot. Although you'll get a better overall compositional change eating good foods regularly, the right supplements at the right time can make a big difference in recovery and making progress. But again, they're supplements, not necessities, though they can be a very useful tool when you're caught short and need to eat but don't have any food available. However, they're not to be thought of as a meal replacement, only as something that can help in times of need.

Think of it this way. If you buy a Sunday paper, you buy it for the news: the front page, the sport, all the normal things you'd expect. There's always a supplement with the paper: financial, housing, TV. But it wouldn't ruin your enjoyment of reading the Sunday paper if they weren't there. You wouldn't stop thinking of it as a Sunday paper if they *weren't* there, but somehow they just add to the whole Sunday paper experience and round it off nicely, making it better overall. The same is true of supplements.

Supplements aren't something I'd force down someone's throat – after all, they're meant to supplement a diet, not replace it, and aren't essential per se. However, there are certain supplements that will help your body function better than it currently does, so you may find some of them worth taking. Furthermore, in terms of the protein requirements laid out in Chapter 4 (3g/kg of bodyweight) it can be very difficult, amid a busy working, training and social lifestyle, to ingest your necessary requirement of protein purely from solid foods. It can also be very expensive to buy good sources of poultry, beef and fish, hence protein shakes are a great addition in many ways. One argument against this is that solid food is far better than 'unnatural protein powders', but this isn't true: solid protein sources haven't been shown to

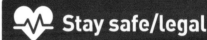

♥ Stay safe/legal

Beyond this book, ensure you do your research on supplements. There are some dangerous products out there that contain ingredients that can be harmful in the wrong mixes/ circumstances. Some of these have hit the press in the past. Only take safe/legal supplements from trustworthy brands.

be superior to liquid sources. At the end of the day, a complete protein containing all the necessary amino acids the human body needs for protein synthesis is a complete protein. There's no real difference other than absorption/digestion rates. Furthermore, protein shakes are derived from whole foods. In fact breast milk is 70% whey protein.

To supplement or not to supplement?

Most people fall into one of three categories:

1 Those who have never taken any supplements, be it protein shakes, fat-burners or energy boosters, and say they 'don't believe in supplements'.

2 Those who religiously use supplements to boost their training, whether they see the benefit or not.

3 Those who occasionally get a pre-made protein shake post-workout or sometimes have a sugary sports drink before or after a hard CV session, ad hoc.

Does one of these sound familiar? I thought so. Let's take each 'type' separately.

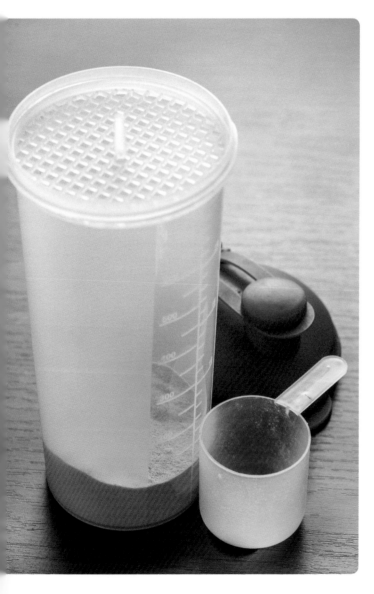

1 The 'no supplements' person

Ladies, don't take this the wrong way, but it's usually you girls who fall into this category. The thought process is that bodybuilders take supplements, so if you even try it then tomorrow you'll wake up looking like a female Arnold Schwarzenegger. Yes, yes, I'm being flippant, but isn't there a little part of you that thinks this?

Just because bodybuilders do something doesn't mean that if you do it you'll suddenly balloon. Put it this way, if I told you Arnold ensures he has seven to eight hours sleep every night, would you suddenly start setting an alarm to get you up after six hours just in case it's the extra sleep causing his excess muscle growth? Again, flippant, but do you see how stupid it is to avoid things just because a certain demographic does them?

I've had female clients worried about eating a higher protein diet (fish, chicken, beef etc) in case they get too big! I understand it's lack of education or understanding that leads to this assumption, but it really is ludicrous. If I or anyone in the fitness industry could create a diet or supplement that can take an average person and turn their physique into something like a pro bodybuilder, do you really think I'd be wasting my time writing this book? No. I'd be promoting my billion-dollar supplement diet, as every young man on the planet would likely want to pay for it.

The only things you absolutely need to avoid are those that are illegal in this country, like steroids and human growth hormones. Supplements aren't in the same category. For one they're legally produced and have to adhere to food standards authorities (at least in the UK). Take MaxiNutrition (the company that I'm an ambassador for, lecture for and openly advise people to use); they're owned by GlaxoSmithKline, the same people that make Sensodyne and Horlicks. MaxiNutrition products are a food, and, even better, unlike other supplement brands MaxiNutrition test EVERY batch that's produced, so when I take it I know that it's been tested to not only provide me with the exact amount of proteins, fats and carbohydrates it says, but also that it hasn't been contaminated with any of the illegal substances that I don't want in my system. Hence England and Lions Rugby and medal-winning brothers the Brownlees and a host of other professional athletes use MaxiNutrition, not to mention supplements themselves.

Do you know what was in that can of Coke you drank last night, or that packet of crisps you ate last weekend? No? See my point?

So, taking a protein supplement doesn't suddenly make you into a *Men's Fitness* cover model – many men wish it would! It takes weeks, months and years of hard work and effort to build muscle; all supplements do is make the hard work pay off that little bit better by providing the necessary nutrients that the body needs to repair, recover and grow more directly.

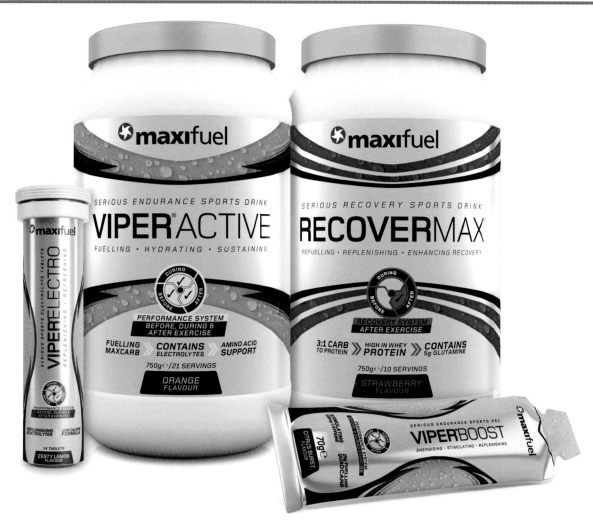

2 The 'take supplements religiously' person

As you can tell from the previous paragraphs, I'm an advocate of supplements. I believe that they're far better than the processed junk foods we get from our supermarkets. Having said that, I'd always recommend real food over supplements if it were a simple choice between one or the other.

So, what of people who religiously take everything the local supplement shop sells or their favourite supplement brand promotes? To be honest, I think they're wasting some of their hard-earned money. Overleaf, I've given the supplements I think are 'should haves' and those I believe are 'nice to haves'. Outside of these I think a lot of products are unnecessary. However, I've also said that everyone is different, so it may be that they'll work for some people and not for others.

What I will say for those of you who have the money and inclination to try every supplement available to make you bigger, stronger, faster and leaner, is *get everything else sorted first*. What do I mean by this? Well, I'm in pretty good shape. I train hard, eat well, supplement sensibly, and have been doing so for some time. If I stopped training altogether and stopped eating sensibly today, yet started taking every 'magic' fat-burner, testosterone booster etc, how long do you think I'd keep

my physique? Not long. So, if you aren't training intensely or following a progressive programme, and are eating really poorly (not enough protein, lots of processed rubbish etc), yet are taking every supplement you can afford, do you really think you'll be able to build a decent physique? Exactly.

Let's make it simple:

- Sort your nutritional needs and buy/prepare/eat sensible foods.
- Follow a structured, progressive training programme as intensely as you can.
- Supplement the above sensibly with whey, omega-3, vit D and a multivitamin.

3 The 'occasional' supplementer

If you do anything half-heartedly, does it ever really work? Put half effort into anything and you get half results. I can hear you now: 'But surely occasionally is better than never at all?' Yes, I'd agree. Occasionally going to the gym is better than never going. You'll be fitter and healthier than someone who doesn't go at all. But we aren't trying to get half results here. I don't work with people who 'half-commit'. Do you want to be the best you can be? Are you going to give this training programme your fullest efforts? Then everything else has to follow.

Protein powders

If you're going to work as hard as you can in the gym, why not give your body every chance of being the best it can be? As I've said before, 'That'll do, will never do'. And I'll say it again: 'That'll do, will never do'.

Firstly, to reiterate, this chapter is about supplements: things that supplement your normal, solid food. Remember, food first wherever possible. There's a place for protein supplementation, and the following explanations aim to give you the ins and outs of the different types of protein powders available.

Where possible, always eat meals that contain beef, poultry, fish, dairy and eggs. As discussed in the nutrition section, this is half the battle to obtaining the physique/figure you want. Some trainers go so far as to simply change someone's diet at first, rather than add exercise, supplements or a calorie deficit, the idea being that a higher protein and far cleaner diet will see fat-loss begin without the other elements. Having said that, protein powders do have some benefits over solid foods, and therefore can be more advantageous at certain times of the day: straight after exercising, being the prime example. I'm therefore going to advocate that as we're only doing this over 12 weeks, and therefore don't have time to change things slowly one at a time, you supplement from the get-go.

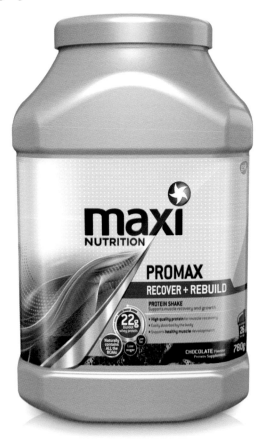

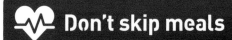

Don't skip meals

Protein powders are meant to supplement your training, not provide meal replacements.

Milk protein

We all drank it from our mothers as babies, most of us drank it from bottles or packets through our formative years and many of us add it to tea or coffee as adults. So what makes up the high-protein drink we know as milk? Two proteins: whey and casein – which are also the two most popular protein powders on the market, with soya now in a close third. Did you know that whey and casein both come from milk? In fact breast milk is 70% whey. In the days before protein powders and supplements, bodybuilders would simply drink milk. I personally drank more milk than water as a kid (or at least, that's how it felt!) – with a nurse for a mother, simple science prevailed, and it certainly doesn't seem to have done me any harm.

Milk itself contains around 8g protein, 8g fat and 11g carbs per 250ml; everything else is simply water. So a glass of milk effectively delivers protein, fats and carbs for your post-workout shake – not bad really. Indeed, if you're ever stuck post-workout and don't believe you can eat for a good few hours due to work or other commitments, a glass of milk could be the answer.

By removing the water and the excess calories from the fat and the carbs (ie lactose, milk's sugar) of cows' milk, supplement companies produce a dry, concentrated protein source. (This isn't just done for the protein benefits that milk can provide, but also because numerous health benefits come from ingesting milk protein, from strengthening the immune system to the obvious performance and physique benefits.) It still contains both casein and whey (around 80/20), so is more beneficial between meals and before bed due to the slow digestion of casein. Whey is digested far faster.

Milk protein can be found as both isolate and concentrate. Concentrate is made by a process called ultrafiltration and leads to a milk protein of around 80%, slightly behind that of a milk protein isolate, with around 85% protein. Again, most of the fats and carbs are removed, with the isolate being slightly further

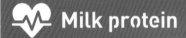

Milk protein

Milk is the protein supplement of the past. There was even a workout programme called 'Squats and milk'.

processed than the concentrate but with no effect on the whey and casein proteins, just less carbs and fats.

Whey protein

From the explanation of milk protein manufacture above, you now understand what whey protein is. However, this still leaves the question as to why it's now the most popular source of protein in sports nutrition. Put simply, whey is the best protein for stimulating protein synthesis within our bodies at a cellular level, and thus for increasing muscle size.

Whey helps increase blood flow and the dilation of blood vessels. Not only has this been shown to help reduce cholesterol and blood pressure, but in terms of sports nutrition it enhances the ability of the body to carry nutrients to the muscles, from amino acids (the bricks from which proteins are made) and proteins, to anabolic hormones like growth hormone and testosterone, not to mention oxygen. All of this not only helps provide more energy and strength during and speedier recovery after training, but also means that the training itself is utilised far more effectively, as the body begins to recover and grow faster and more efficiently afterwards.

Which whey?

Whey comes in three main types from supplement companies: concentrate, isolate and hydrolysate.

Whey concentrate is produced from milk and usually contains 79–80% protein, with some carbs and fats left in. It's a complete protein, meaning it contains all the necessary amino acids that the human body needs to build tissue and muscles. It's produced by microfiltration or ultrafiltration, both of which are actually relatively simple processes. This means that whey concentrate is usually quite cheap, so it's perfect if you're on a budget but keen to get the benefits of protein supplementation.

By means of longer filtration processes such as further microfiltration, cross-flow microfiltration and ion exchange chromatography, supplement companies have been able to produce the purer whey form of isolate. Isolate is around 95% protein or higher, meaning you get more protein for your money, and even more of the carbs and fats are removed. If you can afford it, this is the better form of whey compared to concentrate. I've also found with a few lactose intolerant clients who can't normally eat whey (meaning cheaper whey concentrate usually) that they can take whey isolate without any issues due to the further filtration and removal of carbs (lactose) and fats.

Hydrolysate is whey that's been subjected to hydrolysis. Proteins are made of peptides, peptides are made of amino acids. Although our bodies can take in whole proteins, peptides are absorbed and digested quicker, hence using hydrolysis to break the protein chains into smaller peptides that can be digested faster than isolate. However, due to the further processing this type of protein is usually quite expensive. It isn't necessary, but it could help muscle synthesis and recovery occur more rapidly. If you can afford it use it. If not, stick with a good isolate or a cold-filtered concentrate and spend your extra cash on good solid food.

 Health benefits of whey

Whey has a number of other benefits along with its ability to enhance muscle synthesis. Scientists have shown that whey (or, more specifically, its peptides – the building blocks of protein) inhibit an enzyme called ACE that constricts blood vessels. Whey, therefore, helps to allow greater blood vessel dilation, and lowers blood pressure as well as boosting glutathione, which helps lower total and LDL cholesterol (the bad one). Whey may even help reduce the risk of some cancers.

Why whey?

The question, then, is why do so many people take whey protein compared to others like soya, egg or hemp? Simply put, whey is one of the fastest digesting proteins available. As discussed above, it can be made even quicker by certain processes. Whichever form it's in, it's absorbed into the bloodstream and taken to the muscles faster than the other proteins available. Secondly, whey is very high in the amino acid leucine. Though whey contains all the other amino acids as well, research has shown leucine specifically and directly stimulates protein synthesis, and its higher proportion of leucine therefore renders it a superior protein choice. Lastly, whey is insulinogenic, meaning it boosts insulin levels, and insulin is an anabolic hormone, meaning it helps growth – it literally stimulates muscle protein synthesis.

When to whey?

I'd suggest that the following could be good windows for whey supplementation, depending on your goals and protein requirements:

- First thing in the morning.
- Pre- and post-training.
- As a snack between meals.

 Steroids

Some people seem to associate whey protein supplementation with steroids and bodybuilders. Yes, bodybuilders and steroid users use whey, but they also use cars to drive places. Remember, 70% of breast milk is whey protein and the majority of baby formula milk contains a high percentage of whey! It's simply a great food for growth, repair and health.

Casein protein

As stated earlier, milk is 80% casein and 20% whey. Casein is the insoluble globules of protein that clot in the stomach and can take up to seven hours to digest. This might therefore seem a strange protein to take, considering the manufacture of whey seems to revolve around more and more expensive ways to make it digest faster. However, we're now working at the opposite end of the scale. Casein and its slow absorption rate can help to prevent catabolism – the breakdown of muscle protein by the body for fuel, especially during extended periods without food. This has led to casein becoming a favourite pre-bed supplement within the physique world, to provide the body with a trickle-feed of protein and amino acids overnight to aid recovery, protein synthesis and growth, not to mention minimising muscle breakdown.

Research has also shown that casein can be as effective as whey at stimulating protein synthesis post-training, which isn't surprising really when we remember that old-school bodybuilders would just drink milk! Further studies have shown that people taking casein and whey post-workout demonstrate more muscle growth than those just taking whey, due to the different absorption rates of the two.

Which casein?

Casein protein comes in three forms: micellar casein, caseinate and casein protein hydrolysate.

Micellar casein is casein in its simplest form, and is made using ultrafiltration and then microfiltration to remove the whey, fat and lactose from milk. Despite the processing, the casein still forms micelles (globules) when made into a shake. This can annoy users, as it seems as if it's hard to mix, when actually it's of great benefit as it means that the protein is even slower to digest.

Caseinates come in turn in three forms: calcium caseinate, potassium caseinate and sodium caseinate, which are made by adding either calcium, potassium or sodium respectively. Caseinates usually contain around 90% protein and are the most soluble form of casein. This means they mix better as a shake. However, this also means they digest faster in the stomach – still slower than whey, but faster than micellar casein.

Like whey hydrolysate, casein hydrolysate is pre-digested to make shorter peptides of the casein protein. These digest faster in the stomach, meaning this protein is better pre- or post-workout like whey, rather than before bed like micellar casein. Personally, I'd recommend sticking to whey pre-/post-training, as it'll be cheaper, and stick to casein before bed.

Why casein?

Casein is a slower-digesting protein than whey due to its casein micelles or globules. This makes it a very useful protein before bed, or at times when you'll find it hard to eat over a number of hours and consequently a slow drip-feed of amino acids, due to the slower digestion of casein, is useful. Studies have also shown that taking whey and casein post-workout can increase muscle protein synthesis post-workout compared to just taking whey itself.

When casein?

Taking casein at the following times can reap its slow digestive benefits:

- Before bed.
- Post-workout with whey.
- Before long periods without eating (due to work or endurance activities).

Other protein powders

I'd recommend you use whey and casein proteins because they're simple, can be relatively cheap and provide all the necessary qualities you need to accompany the regular food you eat. However, there are other alternatives, such as:

Beef protein

Beef protein is essentially steak with everything else removed (fat, cholesterol etc), leaving just the protein (amino acids) and the creatine (energy stores in muscle). Beef protein isolate hydrolysed is the most common form, as the protein is pre-digested (as hydrolysed whey is), thus making it digest faster in the stomach. Beef protein is very high protein, often around 99%.

Why beef?

Beef protein contains a high dose of vitamins A, B and D, but above all it's a great alternative for those with dairy or lactose intolerance. It's fast digesting, like whey, but with creatine occurring naturally as an added bonus.

When beef?

- First thing in the morning.
- Pre- and post-workout.
- Between meals.

Egg-white protein

Egg-white protein is recognised as one of the highest quality proteins around. The albumen (egg white) has a very good amino acid make-up, is high in BCAAs (branch chain amino acids) – the true building blocks of proteins – and is very easy for the human body to digest.

The high proportion of BCAAs in egg-white protein means it's proportionally better at helping protein synthesis than other proteins; in fact research has shown that it has similar effects on protein synthesis stimulation to milk protein. Egg-white protein is put through a pasteurisation process to ensure salmonella isn't an issue when being manufactured.

Why egg-white?

Egg-white protein is high in arginine levels. Arginine is an amino acid that has two huge benefits. Firstly arginine can boost natural growth hormone levels. GH, for instance, is a hormone that has a host of benefits, from enhancing muscle growth, increasing new protein synthesis, muscle recovery/repair and metabolism of body fat, to improved sleep pattern, more energy, stronger bones and improved sexual performance. Arginine also stimulates nitric oxide (NO) production. NO is a vasodilator, meaning it increases blood flow to muscles, ensuring that a higher level of oxygen, nutrients and anabolic hormones make it to the muscles, therefore leading to greater muscle growth and improved recovery post-training.

Egg-white is faster digesting than casein, but slower than whey. It's therefore good both for encouraging protein synthesis and for preventing muscle breakdown: a pretty complete protein.

Egg-white protein is again a good alternative for lactose/dairy intolerant people, and like whey it's low in carbs and fats so a good choice in terms of protein powder. Lastly, for those that don't like eggs it's a great way to still benefit from them without actually eating them!

When egg-white?
With its varied qualities, egg can be a useful protein to utilise if you only want to take one with you or if you're dairy intolerant.

- Post-workout.
- Between meals.
- Before bed.

Soy protein
Soy protein is the most popular of plant proteins. However, it's far more popular with women than men, as a big misconception is that because it contains phytoestrogens (plant chemicals that have oestrogen-like properties) it lowers testosterone and raises oestrogen levels. Multiple studies have shown that this is *not* the case. Researchers conclude that soy doesn't alter testosterone concentrations in men whatsoever. Furthermore, a study found that when male bodybuilders supplemented twice daily with either soy protein concentrate powder, soy protein isolate powder, a soy/whey protein powder blend or a whey protein isolate powder during a 12-week weight-training study, all increased muscle mass similarly, regardless of what protein they were taking.

Why soy?
Soy has benefits that whey and other protein powders do not: it

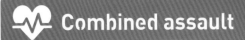

Combined assault
Most recent research has confirmed that taking a protein powder containing whey, casein and soy increases muscle protein synthesis better than either does alone.

Taste of success
When following a different nutrition strategy and training intensely, your protein supplement shakes can be a real 'look-forward', so choose a flavour you like and it can become a helping hand in a completely unexpected way.

can raise GH levels, probably due to its high arginine and lysine content, as well as possibly enhance better muscle recovery due to better antioxidant protection following exercise.

When soy?
10g of soy protein isolate or concentrate post-workout, with whey and casein, seems most beneficial for all. However, for dairy intolerant or vegetarians as your only protein powder:

- Post-workout.
- Between meals.
- Before bed.

Hemp protein
Two proteins make up hemp protein: albumin, which is around 35%, and edestin, which is the other 65%. Due to the make-up of hemp proteins, most are only around 50% protein, but that 50% is arginine and BCAA rich, as well as a very good source of fibre and essential fatty acids.

Pea, brown rice and potato protein powders also exist, but again, I think there are better options, as their percentage of protein isn't particularly high. But if these fit your life choices, they're better than nothing.

That's about it for protein supplementation. In my opinion, when trying to transform your physique protein is probably the most important supplement: not only does it help you get enough protein into the body (up to 2.5–3g/kg of your body weight, remember), which can be tough to do with whole food, but it also ensures a fast-digesting protein gets into the body straight after exercise, and thus to the muscles to aid recovery, switch on protein synthesis, stop catabolism and enhance anabolism.

Whey isolate and casein are the protein choices I personally recommend, unless a client has a dairy intolerance (and is still affected by whey isolate) or is vegan/vegetarian. I personally take whey first thing, pre-training and post-training with a little casein and soya. I have casein before bed as well.

As with anything, it's good to vary, so I don't recommend anyone keeps using exactly the same flavour, brand or type all the time. Look for deals, try different things and work out what works best for you. Variation is key, but don't forget: quality first.

Other supplements

Beyond whey protein, which, as I've said, I believe to be of real benefit to someone trying to change their physique while maintaining their sanity and normal lifestyle (to a point), the following are the other supplements I recommend:

Should-haves

Multivitamin

A good multivitamin from a quality manufacturer can help keep all the necessary bodily functions working properly, especially the immune system, which can become compromised when you drastically change your diet and training regime. Sportsvitamins from MaxiNutrition are my personal choice, but I've also heard great things about Woods supplements. You want your multivit to contain the RDA, or as close to it as possible, of each of its components.

Where possible, get a multivitamin that doesn't contain calcium. Calcium can interfere with the absorption of other minerals, such as zinc and magnesium, so supplementing calcium separately can be the best bet. If you take in sufficient dairy, you may not need to add extra calcium at all. Lastly, zinc and magnesium can be more beneficial when supplemented separately in the form of ZMA, so don't worry too much if your multivit doesn't contain them. Zinc is something that can boost natural testosterone levels, and magnesium has a host of benefits, particularly in helping you to sleep soundly.

Multivits are best taken in the morning.

Vitamin C

Although scurvy isn't as prevalent as it used to be, vitamin C does have a host of other benefits, including helping to rid the body of free radicals as well as boosting the immune system. As vit C is a water-soluble vitamin it's lost in sweating, so as you're going to be undertaking an intense training regime you're likely to require a little more than previously.

A good dose is 500–1,000mg once or twice a day, best taken in the morning or, as many coaches recommend, post-training.

Vitamin D

Although we can 'create' this vitamin when exposed to sunlight, most of us cover up our skin and aren't fortunate enough to live in countries with a good level of sunlight 365 days a year. Therefore, vitamin D supplementation is critical, as it helps with general health, physique and performance, as well as utilisation of minerals like calcium and phosphorous. It aids fat loss, testosterone levels, bone health and mood.

2,000–6,000 IU per day is sufficient, and again is best taken in the morning.

Omega-3 fish oils

The fatty acids eicosapentaenoic acid (EPA) and docosahexaenoic acid (DHA) are the two omega-3 fats that provide all the health, muscle-building and fat-loss benefits of the ever-popular omega-3 supplements. Omega-3s provide numerous health benefits, from helping with fat metabolism to aiding immune health, and are even thought to play an important role in reducing inflammation throughout the body.

Other omega fatty acids include omega-6 and omega-9. Omega-6 fats are commonly found in vegetable oils, so we humans in the Western world are rarely deficient in them. Omega-6s are essential, yet they can become unhealthy when the ratio of omega-6 to omega-3 fats gets higher than 4:1. Eating a diet that's higher than this ratio can prevent optimal muscle recovery and growth, as well as inhibit fat loss – not what you want during your training process. More importantly, a prolonged imbalance could lead to heart disease, cancer, asthma, arthritis and depression. With a ratio of omega-6 to omega-3 fats closer to 1:1 the risk of these diseases is significantly reduced and muscle recovery, growth and fat loss are all greatly enhanced. Simply put, there's no need to supplement with omega-6 fats.

Omega-9 fatty acids aren't essential fats like the 3s and 6s. The human body can produce omega-9 fatty acids on its own. Furthermore, omega-9 fats are in olive oil, and any healthy individual should be cooking with coconut oil and putting olive oil on their food anyway, meaning you'll be getting adequate amounts of omega-9 fats. So again, there's no need to supplement with omega-9 fats.

A lot of supplements for omegas are omega-3-6-9 mixtures. The downside of these is that, as explained, we don't really need to supplement 6 and 9, and as these mixtures only contain 10–20% of the amount of omega-3 fats as fish oil supplements, you're really wasting your time and money, as you won't get ample amounts of omega-3 and you'd be supplementing with omega-6 fats and omega-9 fats which you don't really need.

Supplement with 2–3g of omega-3 fish oil once or twice a day. Ideally this will give you 1,500mg of DHA per day. Your fish oil supplement will tell you how much DHA, as well as EPA, is in

 Something fishy

If you eat one to two portions of oily fish a day, you arguably don't need an omega-3 supplement; however, there is no research to suggest too much is bad, so it won't hurt to supplement as well as ingest via food.

each capsule. By ensuring 1,500mg of DHA you'll get enough EPA too, as it's in higher amounts than DHA in fish oil.

ZMA or magnesium spray

ZMA is a zinc, magnesium and vitamin B6 complex that's common within the fitness industry. Taking ZMA 30–60 minutes before bed can help increase sleep quality and keep your testosterone levels and muscle strength up. Zinc has been shown to have positive effects on testosterone, whereas magnesium has been proven to help sound sleep, and since recovery is so important for fat loss and muscle gain this is turn will have a huge effect on your compositional changes.

As stated, ZMA provides B6. In general the B vitamins can be low in those who train, as they're lost in sweat. Your multivitamin should contain all necessary B vitamins, but a ZMA will bolster your B6.

Personally, I've had trouble sleeping over the years. I think I became a very light sleeper during Royal Marine training and have never truly recovered from it. While writing books I tend to have trouble sleeping while coming up with ideas and as the deadline approaches, being unable to switch off. However, I've found that a separate magnesium spray (sprayed on to the soft skin under the elbow and behind the knee) has worked wonders. I use BetterYou, who also do magnesium salts for baths, which friends have told me really help with muscle aches.

Creatine

Creatine has been a controversial supplement for no real reason. Personally I advise you to have it. It's naturally occurring in the muscles of animals and humans and is involved in one of the three energy systems that allow us to function. There are now a few hundred studies on the effectiveness and safety of creatine. Research has shown that it's both extremely effective and also very safe, and leads to long-term increases in muscle growth and strength through a number of different mechanisms. Research has also shown that worries over dehydration, muscle cramps or muscle injuries are completely unfounded. Creatine comes in a few forms, but basic creatine monohydrate is fine.

Take 2–5g of creatine with your pre- and post-workout shake. If only one, then just your post-workout. On rest days, take one dose of creatine at some point. Some people believe a loading phase (ie 5–7 days of a much larger dose, around 20g – thought to fully saturate the muscle's stores – before moving on to the maintenance phase of 2–5g) is necessary. You can do this, but it isn't necessarily critical.

Nice-to-haves

Beta-alanine

Although ingested naturally from meat sources such as beef and poultry, beta-alanine can also be supplemented for added benefits. It's taken up by the muscle fibres and combines with the amino acid histidine to form the dipeptide (two amino acid

protein) carnosine. It's carnosine that provides all the benefits that studies have shown are associated with beta-alanine: greater strength and power, better endurance, greater fat loss and more muscle growth.

2–3g of beta-alanine before and after training is optimal. However, it does have a side-effect of making the skin tingle or itch, which although it's a novelty and perhaps useful pre-training, can be a little off-putting when you return to work, so carefully test the dosage and timing (this is harmless and nothing to worry about). I've seen lots of friends and clients rubbing their hairlines mid-session, much to my amusement! You have been warned.

CLA

Conjugated linoleic acid is a naturally occurring fatty acid found in meat and dairy. Research has shown that CLA not only helps lower body fat considerably, but can also increase muscle mass and strength. It's also been credited with reducing the risk of certain cancers. Effects take place over a lengthy time period, usually around three months, so if you decide to supplement with CLA do so from the start. Take one capsule two or three times a day.

Green tea extract

Green tea contains catechins, including EGCG, which makes green tea very thermogenic. The reason for this is that EGCG inhibits the enzyme that breaks down noradrenalin, which usually regulates your metabolic rate and fat burning. It also contains caffeine so can replace tea or coffee. Joint healing and lower risk of certain cancers has also been attributed to green tea. Research has shown that extract is better absorbed than the tea, so taking two or three 500mg caps a day, before meals, would be most beneficial.

⏱ Conclusion

There are other supplements that I take or have taken, from BCAAs and arginine to HMB, D-aspartic acid and glutamine etc. These all have different benefits, and have undergone research that supports their credibility. However, this transformation book is intended to provide basic recommendations regarding supplements and an outline of their benefits, without either confusing you or breaking the bank. Therefore although some of the supplements mentioned could be useful, I believe you'll get good results without them. Once you've completed your body transformation programme you then have the option of trying them later to see if they make a significant difference.

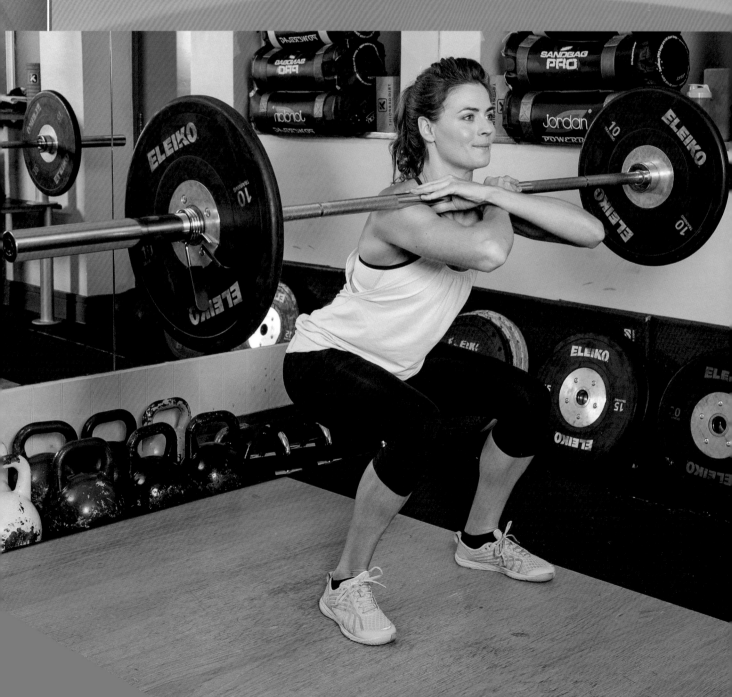

CHAPTER 6
TRAINING PLAN

The following chapter includes the complete training programme you'll be following, from week 1 to week 12, across the five microcycles. Simply put, eat as instructed in the nutrition chapter and follow this programme to the letter (ensuring your weights are at an adequate level to make the sessions intense, take you to a failure point, and are progressed from the previous session), and you'll experience dramatic changes, both physical and mental.

Before we get to the programme itself, it may help you if I provide a few explanations as to why the programme is designed in the way that it is.

Periodisation

Professional athletes, bodybuilders and sports players will have their training 'periodised'. What this means is that after a set period of time they'll change from one style of training to another. The original concept behind periodisation was to concentrate on different aspects that the athlete would need to successfully compete at his or her chosen sport. For example, a boxer preparing for a fight in four months' time might do a strength and conditioning programme consisting of the following:

- One month of strength work (low reps, heavy weight) and LISS for general fitness.
- One month of hypertrophy work (8–12 reps, medium weights) and HIIT to help growth.
- One month of endurance work (high reps, light weight) and LISS for bout endurance.
- One month of stamina and weight-loss, so circuits, complexes and LISS and HIIT for all-round fitness.

The added bonus with periodising training is that it forces the body to change and adapt. The human body is a very adaptable organism. This is a good thing, but in terms of training it can be a bad thing. It means you can't adopt one type of training and stick with it: your body will simply adapt and be comfortable. We therefore try to reduce this adaptation by continually progressing – adding weight, adding reps or sets, reducing rest times etc. However, before we know it a simple, set training programme can still become stale and stagnated, and we need a new challenge. Periodisation offers this, but over 4–12 months, as an athlete prepares for a big event or the climax of the season.

Microcycles

So, how can we utilise periodisation to get the best out of it for you and your body transformation over a shorter period, like 12 weeks? Simple. We utilise the general idea of periodisation but on a much smaller scale. Instead of months we look at weeks or 'microcycles'. These microcycles allow us to change the training throughout your 12-week journey to continually keep the body guessing: to force adaptations, increase muscle and strength gains, keep intensity high and thus burn body fat. An added bonus is that it'll keep you interested and stop you getting bored and giving up! Yes, doing the same session for a month in a linear fashion, keeping everything the same but increasing the weight, will lead to changes, but research has shown that the gains aren't as pronounced as using the format laid out in this chapter: changing the reps, weights, exercises, tempo etc, but in a logical, specific manner to maximise fitness, fat loss and muscle gain. 'Logical variety' is the term I like to use.

For example, in week one you'll be working at higher reps and lower weights. This is simply to get the whole body working together and not applying too much weight if you're not used to it. In week two your reps will go down, rest will come down, and of course the weights will need to increase in turn. This should add some strength but still not be too intense, so as to ease you in. For week three (microcycle 2), reps will jump again to 12–15, weights will drop and so will rest. This cycle of upping and downing reps and weights continues before returning to a rep range that you've done before – but don't you dare use the same weight as three or four weeks ago for those reps! You should've become stronger, so you need to use a bigger weight for the same exercise, doing your best to match the reps from before. On top of changing reps, tempo changes, rest times and of course exercise selection, you'll pair exercises as the weeks go by to form supersets, you'll maximise time and improve your exercise intensity, thus burning more body fat.

Change to succeed

One of the most common mistakes people make in the gym is to follow the same programme and lift the same weights, week in, week out, expecting to see change. If you do the same things, you'll see the same you. But if you change the programme, change the weights, change the reps, then you'll see a different you.

This may sound complicated, but it really isn't. The idea is simply to keep your body guessing and to keep it interesting for you, without a host of weird and wonderful exercises that I believe have been the downfall of other such programmes in the past. Simplicity, after all, can be a godsend. Remember the Marines' acronym KISS: keep it simple, stupid.

Success

For you to succeed at this, all you have to do is work *as hard as you can*. As was discussed in Chapter 3, you have to train with intensity. If you aren't struggling towards the end of the given rep range, then the weight isn't heavy enough. You MUST change up to a heavier weight or you'll be wasting your training session, and you'll be that little bit behind the point that you *should* have reached. Having said that, the reason you'll get good muscle gains from this type of training is because you'll not only be changing the rep ranges weekly, but also because you keep the same weight on each exercise for all sets in a session, while still making yourself complete the given reps, drop sets or rest/pause sets. Unless you can't complete the minimum reps in set 1, don't be tempted to drop the weight (barring injury etc): stick with it, work intensely and let the programme do its magic.

Work consistently for each session, each week, and you'll get the results. It's your new body, your health and your change. It's up to you. I've given you the tools. You have to do the work.

Splits

Some of you will have heard of splits, some of you won't. In short, you can split up your body or muscle groups in different

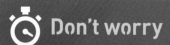

Don't worry

Try not to worry or second-guess things. Take each day as it comes, approach it as if it's your last and make it count. If you do that, then by the end of 12 weeks you'll see the difference.

ways to train them. How you split is quite an individual thing; some people like to train their whole body in one, others like to train legs all on their own, or train their biceps with their chest or any other variation that works for them.

How you split your training often depends on several things:

- How experienced or new you are to training.
- How many times a week you wish to train.
- How long it takes you to recover.
- What you did for your last training cycle.
- How intense your training is.
- How much volume (amounts of sets and reps) per session.
- Personal preferences.
- Personal weaknesses.

In this programme we'll be starting as if you're untrained and inexperienced. This is therefore a good starting point for anyone – beginner, novice, returnee from injury or prolonged absence or even someone with experience. We'll be starting with complete body training in microcycle 1, then in microcycle 2 we'll be splitting upper and lower body up, and from microcycle 3 onwards we'll be grouping different muscle groups for different sessions. For example, you'll do push and pull days in microcycle 3, whereas microcycle 4 will see good old back and biceps grouped together along with chest and triceps – the bodybuilders' favourite. To reiterate, the variation is done on purpose, to keep the body guessing, help you overcome plateaus and stop you getting bored. Also, changing which muscles work with which will hopefully help you overcome muscle imbalances or pre-fatigue if certain muscles dominate certain movements.

All you have to do is worry about each day's training session, work hard, eat as best you can by the guidelines and get enough sleep. The rest will take care of itself.

Rest

We've already discussed rest in the exercise fundamentals chapter, but to reiterate, rest days and rest times are there for a reason. Follow them. If it says rest 60 seconds, then rest 60 seconds. If you start after 50 seconds you'll either fail too early or your weights are too light. Equally, don't wait for 90 seconds because you're talking to someone; you need to be consistent, and the overall effect of the programme that day is important, not just that set. The culmination is imperative.

Lastly, a rest day is a rest day for a reason. Don't go to the gym. Don't go to a spin class. Don't go for a yoga class. Rest – perhaps have a massage or a stretch, but no more. Be confident in what you did yesterday at the gym and let your body change as it rests. Rest stands for Recovery Equals Successful Training. If you train on your rest days you'll burn out, get injured, or simply not have enough energy later in the programme to do what's asked of you.

Resistance training

The resistance training sessions are split across 12 weeks and 5 'microcycles'. The microcycles serve to group together similar sessions or styles of session, to allow you to see progress despite the constant changing of the training which ensures progressive overload and variation. Varying and progressively overloading key compound exercises and some isolation exercises within a hypertrophy specific rep range of 6–15 reps (not 30–50, ladies), combined with a good nutritional plan, will ensure that you get the results you desire, and that's what the training programme reflects.

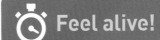

Feel alive!

Remember, training by itself isn't enough. Too many gym-goers forget or ignore this fact.

NB: Using the training protocols outlined in previous chapters, you must ensure you're training intensely and hitting failure within the 6–15 reps designated, in order to guarantee results.

Cardio training

Cardiovascular training is also included, starting with interval training and changing to more recognisable steady state CV training towards the end. This is simply because interval training is known to yield better results for fat burning, yet is also more degrading/fatiguing long-term. Therefore as the resistance training increases in volume and intensity we decrease high-intensity cardiovascular intervals with less intense steady state sessions. Cardiovascular training is usually the training that most people focus on when trying to obtain a better physique or figure, yet it will actually only make up a small proportion of the training. Like the resistance training, it needs to be progressive (ie get harder) and intense (you need to be pushing yourself).

As discussed earlier, we'll be using two types of cardiovascular training: HIIT (high intensity interval training) and LISS (low intensity steady state).

HIIT

HIIT training has recently become the favoured method for reducing body fat. It's been shown to induce a larger loss on a minute per minute basis than LISS. However, it's intense and tough, and therefore when done frequently can cause injury and burnout. This is especially true if you're also on a calorie deficit and doing exceptionally intense and demanding resistance sessions, as you will be on this programme. Therefore we'll utilise HIIT once a week early on in your programme when the resistance training isn't so intense or so frequent. Then concentrate on LISS sessions later in the programme so that intense resistance sessions can remain the focus.

LISS

LISS is a great way of reducing body fat alongside a hard/intense resistance programme. Many physique competitors prefer LISS as it accompanies their resistance training and 'diets' well, since

it's only necessary to train at low to moderate intensity and fat loss still occurs. The problem is, too many people who don't know any better rely on LISS alone, with no resistance training or nutrition plan, and therefore see very little change. Disheartened with their efforts in the gym, they give up, believing genetics has them beat. Not so.

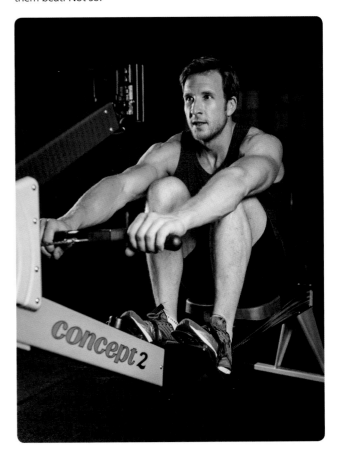

Alongside a good resistance programme, LISS won't burn you out, and thus for most people works alongside weight training better than HIIT. Personally, I still prefer HIIT, but that may be my background as a 400m runner! It's true that LISS can be performed more frequently than HIIT without eating into recovery, which is too easily compromised during a 12-week training programme where your training volume is likely to be far higher than you've experienced before. LISS can also be a great way to start the day, especially in the summer, and particularly if you're a fan of running and don't want to lose this training in favour of the much-needed resistance work. Do be aware, though, that many physique competitors still get 'cover model' lean without performing any LISS at all. Diet and resistance training alone is sufficient if both are followed properly.

Fasted HIIT or LISS

Something which many of you will have heard about, or indeed tried, is 'fasted cardio', *ie* cardiovascular training when you have little or no stored 'food' in your system (you haven't eaten), the idea being that your body will more readily use increased amounts of body fat for energy.

Most people therefore do this first thing in the morning before eating, as they'll have 'starved' overnight. Despite having done this myself, there's still debate as to whether it's necessary or more beneficial. Recent research suggests that although more fat is burned when doing cardio fasted, it could encourage breakdown of the muscle tissue you're so painstakingly trying to build. Therefore, considering that fasted cardio may make little or no difference to fat loss compared with fed cardio, but could lead to more muscle breakdown, it may be safer to do cardio fed. A recent study at a British university stated that you could do LISS (not HIIT, as it's too intense and will cause muscle breakdown) fasted or fed, but if doing it fed you should try to avoid carbohydrate and eat only protein where possible.

I'm personally an advocate for morning cardio with resistance training in the afternoon or evening, as it suits my lifestyle and I feel it works for me. However, the mistake many trainers make is

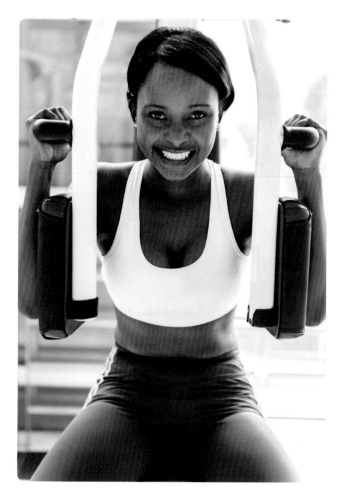

assuming that what works for them also works for their clients. Unfortunately we're all different, and what works for me may not work for you. Therefore if you wanted to try it fasted you could certainly give it a go. If you don't fancy it, then a protein shake before cardio training is a perfect solution, with a good balanced meal on completion. Again, although not necessarily right for everyone, this is my preferred LISS training: protein shake, LISS, shower, breakfast, then my day.

Abs and spot reduction?

Many of you will see the emergence of a six-pack as the holy grail of your body transformation. It seems to be the marker by which everyone judges a successful change. With that in mind, I just want to reiterate that you can't get a six-pack by doing endless sit-ups. It doesn't work that way. To see your six-pack, we need to lower your body fat, simple as that, and to lower your body fat we need to ensure you have a good exercise programme accompanied by a sensible and considered calorific deficit-based nutrition plan. Basically, everything we've set out to do in this book. Again, we're not going to include endless abs exercises at the end of each

session to get your six-pack; they won't help and won't get you there any quicker. There are far better things we could utilise that time for, like preparing the next day's food.

If you follow this plan, then depending on your efforts (the amount of intensity you put in) and your ability to stay focused, you should get as close to a six-pack appearing as you've ever had. If it doesn't quite get there, take a week off and repeat weeks 1–12 or 5–12. There's no reason why you can't repeat the programme. If you'd rather do something different, see Chapter 10, in which I outline 'the next step'.

The transformation programme

The idea behind this programme is that everyone undertaking it will perform all 12 weeks from start to finish, never missing a session and following each to the tee. Coupled with a high protein diet giving a calorific deficit, that includes a good source of healthy fats and sensible carbohydrate, this will yield dramatic changes in your physique.

However, I appreciate that some people may not wish to undertake all 12 weeks for whatever reason (a wedding in six weeks, already relatively lean, holiday in a month etc), therefore I've put together the following guidelines for only completing part of the programme.

To reiterate, I advise everyone to do all 12 weeks, but if you must cut it short diet is still paramount, and intensity of each session even more important (as you'll do less).

Completing last four weeks only (weeks 9–12)
Advanced trainers only, who already train regularly and are used to following a structured training programme. Body fat should be under 15% for men and under 18% for women.

Completing last eight weeks only (weeks 5–12)
Intermediate trainers who already train regularly, but perhaps not intensely enough, and who don't eat as well as they could. Body fat should be under 18% for men and under 25% for women.

At the opposite end of the spectrum, if over 30% for a man and 35% for a woman, or very new to this type of exercise, doing microcycles 1 and 2 twice, right through, increasing the weights throughout and thus making the whole process 16 weeks, could yield far better results for you.

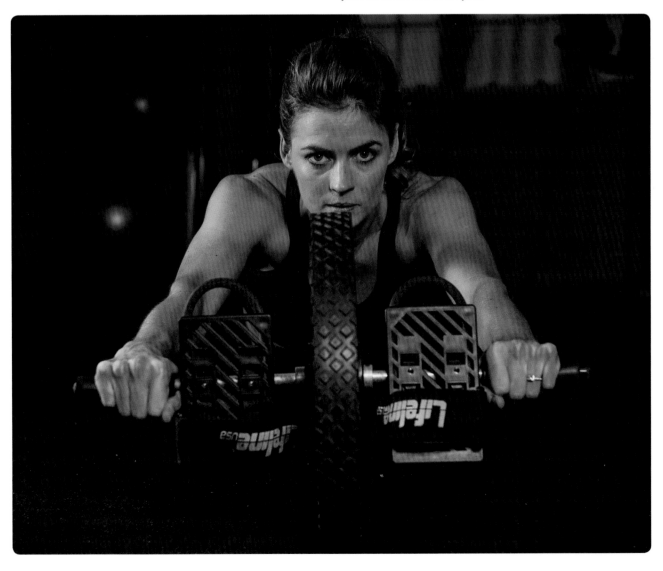

Microcycle 1
WEEK 1

MONDAY

Full body

5 minutes cardio: jog, bike, row.

Mobility.

Dynamic stretch.

Tempo 3010.

90 seconds rest between sets.

Three sets of:

Deadlifts 8–12 reps.

Squats 8–12 reps.

Bench press 8–12 reps.

Chin-ups 4–6 reps or 4–6 reps jump up and eccentric lower or mix of both.

Overhead press 8–12 reps.

Reps.

Abs

Cable abs curls 10–15 reps.

Incline reverse crunch 10–15 reps.

Side-bends with dumbbell 10–15 reps each side.

Finisher

Push press 8–12 reps.

TUESDAY

Rest.

WEDNESDAY

Full body

5 minutes cardio: jog, bike, row.

Mobility.

Dynamic stretch.

Tempo 3010.

90 seconds rest between sets.

Try to increase weights from Monday by 2–2.5kg.

Three sets of:

Chin-ups 4–6 reps or 4–6 reps jump up and eccentric lower or mix of both.

Squats 8–12 reps.

Bench press 8–12 reps.

Deadlifts 8–12 reps.

Overhead press 8–12 reps.

Abs

Cable abs curls 10–15 reps.

Incline reverse crunch 10–15 reps.

Side-bends with dumbbell 10–15 reps each side.

Finisher

Power cleans 8–12 reps.

THURSDAY

Rest.

FRIDAY

Full body

5 minutes cardio: jog, bike, row.

Mobility.

Dynamic stretch.

Tempo 3010.

90 seconds rest between sets.

Try to increase weights from Wednesday by 2–2.5kg.

Three sets of:

Deadlifts 6–10 reps.

Overhead press 6–10 reps.

Chin-ups 4–6 reps or 4–6 reps jump up and eccentric lower or mix of both.

Squats 6–10 reps.

Bench press 6–10 reps.

Abs

Cable abs curl 10–15 reps.

Incline reverse crunch 10–15 reps.

Side-bends with dumbbell 10–15 reps each side.

Finisher

Kettlebell swings 15–20 reps.

SATURDAY

Sprint intervals.

5–10 minute jog.

Dynamic stretch.

6 x 40m sprints.

SUNDAY

Rest.

Deadlifts

▶ Place hands a little wider than shoulder-width apart. Arms should be straight, head up, chest up and out. Extend legs and hips and pushing the feet into the floor. Arms and back remain straight and the bar is kept close to the body. Return the bar to the floor under control, pushing the hips back. Ensure the back is always straight. Repeat.

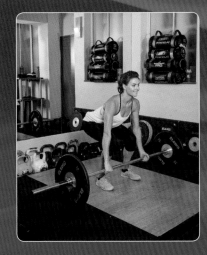 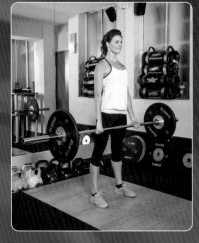

Squats

▶ Take a barbell across the shoulder and grasp to the sides. Stand with shoulder width stance and squat down by bending hips back while allowing knees to bend forward, keeping back straight and knees pointed same direction as feet. Descend until thighs are just past parallel to floor. Extend knees and hips until legs are straight to return to start position. Repeat.

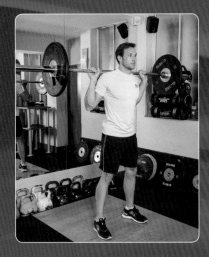 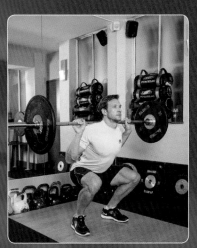

Bench press

▶ While laid back on a bench, a weighted barbell is taken from straight arms (above the chest) to bent arms, just touching the chest, before it is returned to the start position. It is important not to 'bounce' the weight off the chest. Try to keep your upper arm at a 45 degree angle to your body.

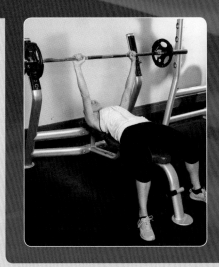 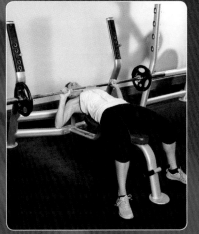

WEEK

1
2
3
4
5
6
7
8
9
10
11
12

Chin-ups

▶ Grasp bar with underhand shoulder-width grip. Pull body up until elbows are to sides and chin over bar. Lower body until arms and shoulders are fully extended. Repeat.

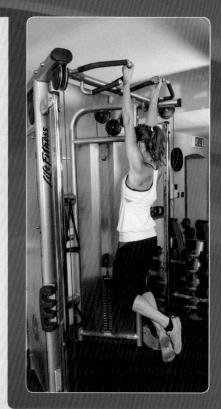
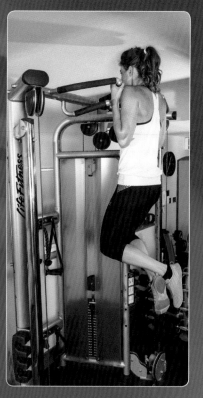

Overhead press

▶ Hold barbell on the top of the chest with a slightly wider than shoulder-width overhand grip at the front of the neck. Press bar upward until arms are extended overhead. Lower to front of neck and repeat.

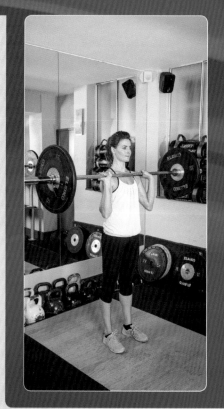
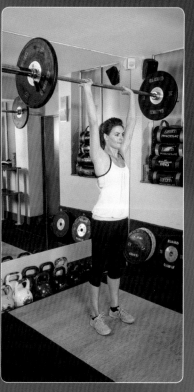

Cable ab curls

▶ Kneel below high pulley holding cable rope attachment with both hands. Place wrists against head. Position hips back and flex hips, allowing resistance on cable pulley to lift torso upward so spine is hyperextended. With hips stationary, flex waist so forehead moves towards floor. Return and repeat.

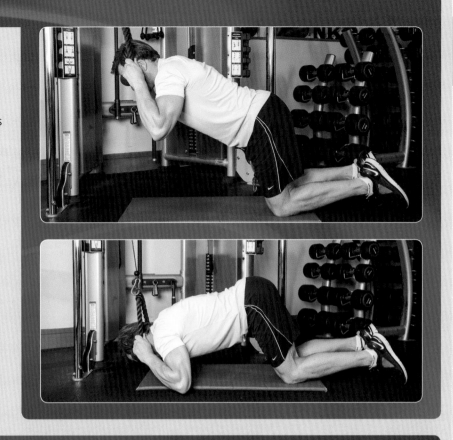

Incline reverse crunch

▶ Using an inclined bench, lie supine holding onto the bench overhead for support. Raise legs by flexing hips while flexing knees until hips are fully flexed. Continue to raise knees toward shoulders by flexing waist, raising hips from bench. Return until waist and hips are extended and repeat.

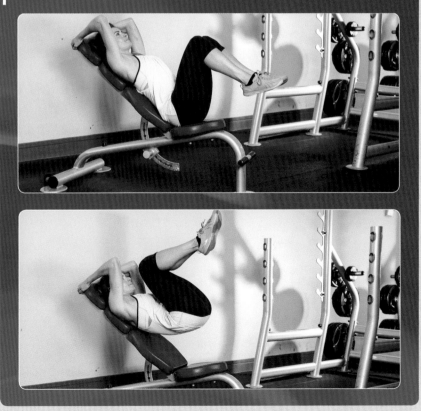

Side bends with dumbbells

▶ Grasp dumbbell with arm straight to side. Bend waist to opposite side of dumbbell until touching the knee area. Lower to opposite side, same distance and repeat. Continue with opposite side.

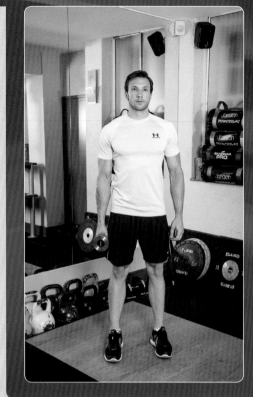
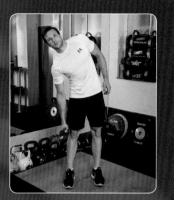
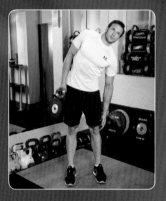

Push press

▶ Either clean a barbell up to the shoulders or take it from a rack onto the shoulders/top of chest with grip slightly wider than shoulder width. Dip body by bending knees, hips and ankles slightly, then explosively drive upward with legs, driving barbell up off shoulders, vigorously extending arms until overhead. Return to shoulders under control and repeat.

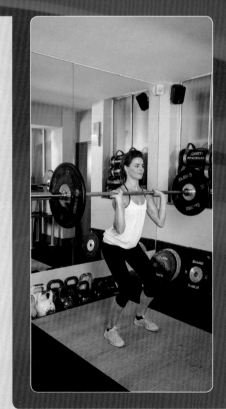
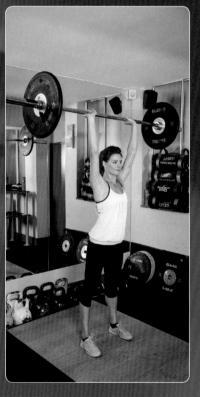

Power clean

▶ Stand over barbell with balls of feet positioned under bar and hip-width apart or slightly wider. Squat down and grip bar with overhand grip slightly wider than shoulder width. Position shoulders over bar with back arched tightly. Arms are straight with elbows pointed along bar. Pull bar up off floor by extending hips and knees. As bar reaches knees, vigorously raise shoulders while keeping barbell close to thighs. When barbell passes mid-thigh, allow it to contact thighs and almost jump upward to extend the body. Shrug shoulders and pull barbell upward with arms, allowing elbows to flex but keeping bar close to body. Aggressively pull body under bar, rotating elbows around bar to allow a catch on shoulders before knees bend lower than 90°. Stand up immediately so thighs are no lower than parallel to floor. Reverse the movement at pace to carefully lower bar to the floor and repeat.

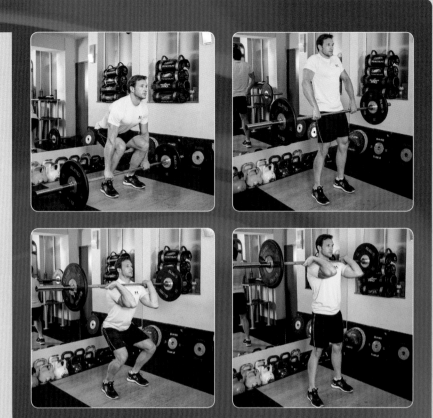

Kettlebell swings

▶ Place the bell in between the legs with handle parallel to the shoulders. Squat down and take hold of the handle, keeping the back straight and head up. Perform a powerful squat, paying particular attention to driving the hips forward (a hip thrust) and squeezing the glutes together. In doing this, momentum allows the bell to come up to around eye level by rotating through the shoulders. As the bell starts to drop (gravity), bend the legs into the squat position again; as the bell comes in between the legs, drive up again and thrust the hips forward. Repeat for a certain number of reps or for a set time.

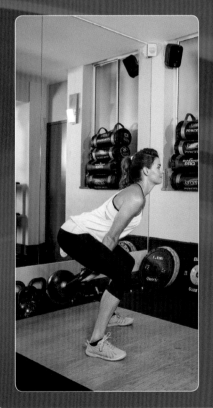
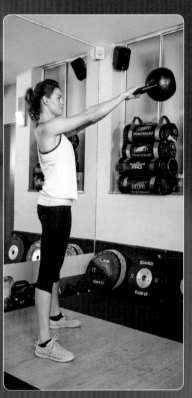

Microcycle 1
WEEK 2

MONDAY

Full body

5 minutes cardio: jog, bike, row.
Mobility.
Dynamic stretch.
Tempo 3010.
2 minutes rest between sets.
Try to increase weights from Monday by 2–2.5kg.
Three sets of:
Squats 6–10 reps.
Deadlifts 6–10 reps.
Overhead press 6–10 reps.
Chin-ups 4–6 reps or 4–6 reps jump up and eccentric lower or mix of both.
Bench press 6–10 reps.

Abs

Cable abs curls 10–15 reps.
Incline reverse crunch 10–15 reps.
Side-bends with Olympic bar 10–15 reps.

TUESDAY

Rest.

WEDNESDAY

Full body

5 minutes cardio: jog, bike, row.
Mobility.
Dynamic stretch.
Tempo 3010.
2 minutes rest between sets.
Try to choose heavy but achievable weights.
Three sets of:
Deadlifts 4–6 reps.
Bench press 4–6 reps.
Squats 4–6 reps.
Overhead press 4–6 reps.
Chin-ups 4–6 reps or 4–6 reps jump up and eccentric lower or mix of both.

Abs

Cable abs curls 10–15 reps.
Incline reverse crunch 10–15 reps.
Side-bends with Olympic bar 10–15 reps.

THURSDAY

Rest.

FRIDAY

Full body

5 minutes cardio: jog, bike, row.
Mobility.
Dynamic stretch.
Tempo 3010.
2 minutes rest between sets.
Try to increase weights from Wednesday by 2–2.5kg.
Three sets of:
Squats 4–6 reps.
Overhead press 4–6 reps.
Chin-ups 4–6 reps or 4–6 reps jump up and eccentric lower or mix of both.
Bench press 4–6 reps.
Deadlifts 4-6 reps.

Abs

Cable abs curls 10–15 reps.
Incline reverse crunch 10–15 reps.
Side bends with Olympic bar 10–15 reps.

SATURDAY

Rest.

SUNDAY

Rest.

Side-bends with Olympic bar

▶ Place an olympic bar across the shoulders/traps and stand with feet around shoulder-width apart. Lean over to one side, controlling the movement with the core. Return to the start position but continue past it to lean in the opposite direction. Repeat.

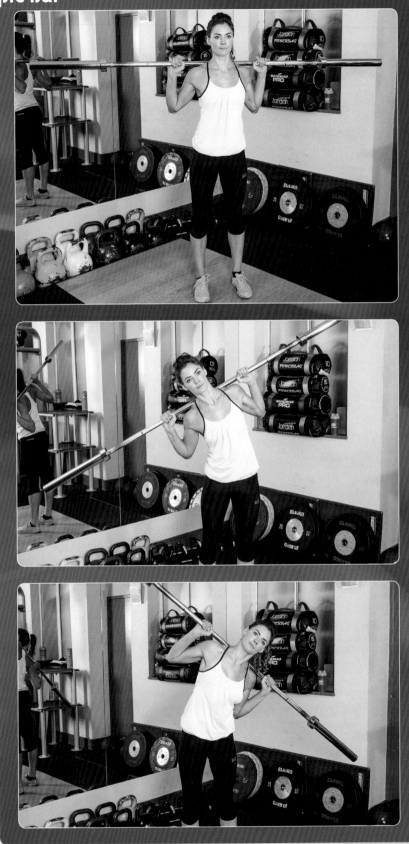

Microcycle 2
WEEK 3

Monday
Upper body
5 minutes cardio: jog, bike, row.
Mobility.
Dynamic stretch.
Tempo 40X0.
90 seconds rest between sets.
Three sets of:
Bench press 12–15 reps.
Pull-ups to failure into inverted row 12–15 reps.
Overhead press 12–15 reps.
Incline dumbbell press 12–15 reps.
Bent-over row 12–15 reps.
Seated dumbbell shoulder press 12–15 reps.
Finisher
Push press 12–15 reps.

Tuesday
Legs and abs
5 minutes cardio: jog, bike, row.
Mobility.
Dynamic stretch.
Tempo 40X0.
90 seconds rest between sets.
Three sets of:
Deadlifts 12–15 reps.
Squats 12–15 reps.
Front squats 12–15 reps.
Straight-leg deadlifts 12–15 reps.
Leg extensions 12–15 reps.
Leg curls 12–15 reps.
Rollouts 6–10 reps.
Incline reverse crunch 8–12 reps.
Sit-ups 8–12 reps.
Finisher
Kettlebell swings 12–15 reps.

Wednesday
Rest.

Thursday
Upper body
5 minutes cardio: jog, bike, row.
Mobility.
Dynamic stretch.
Try to increase weights by 2.5–5kg from Monday.
Tempo 40X0.
90 seconds rest between sets.
Three sets of:
Bench press 8–12 reps.
Pull-ups to failure into inverted row 8–12 reps.
Overhead press 8–12 reps.
Incline dumbbell press 8–12 reps.
Bent-over row 8–12 reps.
Seated dumbbell shoulder press 8–12 reps.
Finisher
Dumbbell snatches 8–12 reps each side.

Friday
Legs and abs
5 minutes cardio: jog, bike, row.
Mobility.
Dynamic stretch.
Try to increase weights by 2.5–5kg from Tuesday.
Tempo 40X0.
90 seconds rest between sets.
Three sets of:
Deadlifts 8–12 reps.
Squats 8–12 reps.
Front squats 8–12 reps.
Straight-leg deadlifts 8–12 reps.
Leg extension 8–12 reps.
Leg curls 8–12 reps.
Rollouts 6–10 reps.
Incline reverse crunch 8–12 reps.
Sit-ups 8–12 reps.
Finisher
Power cleans 8–12 reps.

Saturday
Sprint intervals.
5–10 minute jog.
Dynamic stretch.
8 x 40m sprints.

Sunday
Rest.

Pull-ups

▶ Start with hands just a little more than shoulder-width apart. Hands should be pronated (with the palms turned away). Pull up, bending the elbows and bringing the chin up to the bar. Lower to start position under control. Repeat.

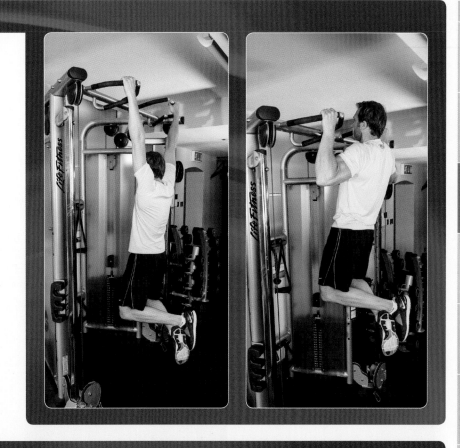

Inverted row

▶ Lie on floor on back under fixed horizontal bar or TRX handles. Grasp bar/handles with overhand grip. Keeping body straight, from ankles to knees to hips to shoulders, pull body up to bar. Return until arms are extended and shoulders are stretched forward. Repeat.

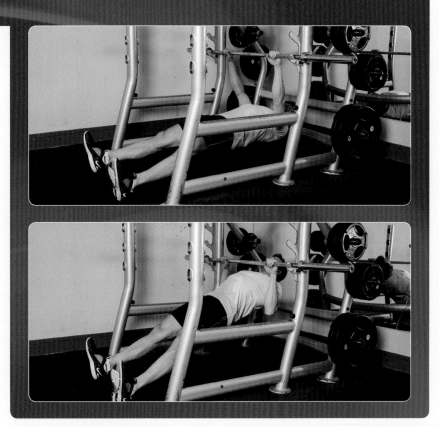

WEEK

1
2
3
4
5
6
7
8
9
10
11
12

Incline dumbbell press

► Lie on incline bench with dumbbells in the hands above the upper chest in an overhand grip. Lower weights to the upper chest, then press until arms are extended. Repeat.

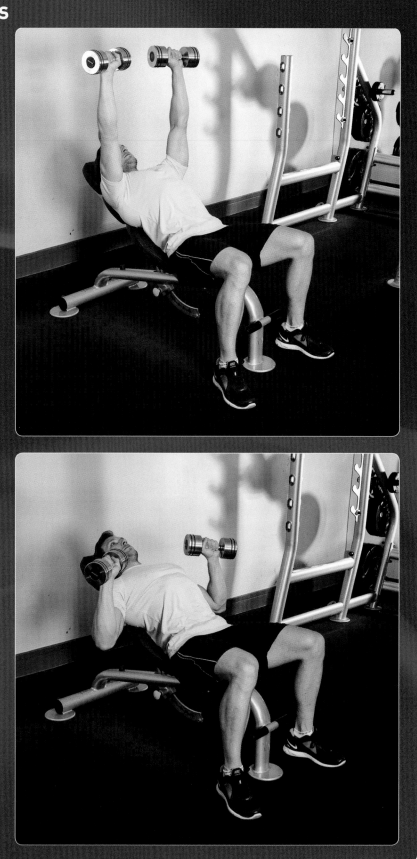

Bent-over row

▶ Hold a barbell with slightly bent knees and a straight back. Use a shoulder-width overhand grip. Pull bar to upper waist (belly button region). Return until arms are extended and shoulders are stretched downward. Repeat.

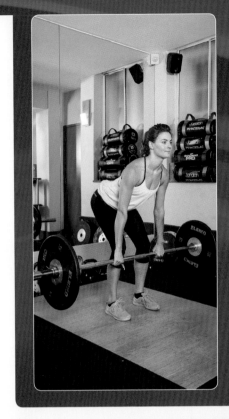
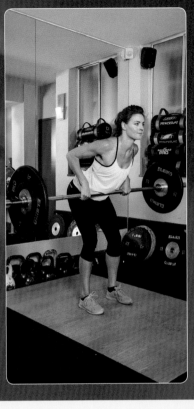

Seated dumbbell shoulder press

▶ Position dumbbells to each side of shoulders with elbows below wrists. Press dumbbells upward until arms are extended overhead. Lower to sides of shoulders into start position and repeat.

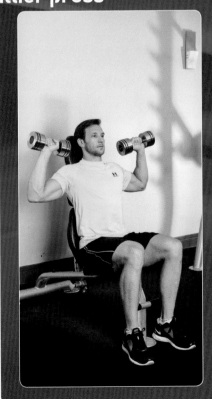
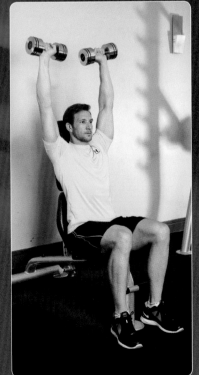

Front squats

▶ Take a barbell onto the upper chest either by crossing arms and placing hands on top of the barbell or with an open grasp and elbows high. Either way, ensure upper arms are parallel to floor. Squat down by bending hips back while allowing knees to bend forward, keeping back straight and knees pointed in same direction as feet. Descend until thighs are just past parallel. Extend knees and hips until legs are straight. Return and repeat.

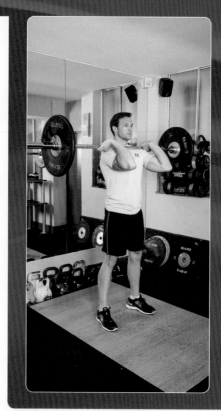
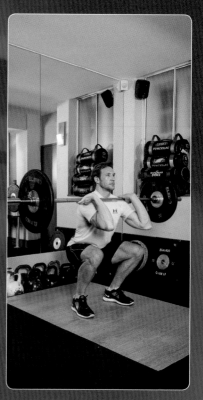

Straight-leg deadlifts

▶ Stand with shoulder-width or narrower stance with feet flat beneath bar. Bend knees and bend over with lower back straight. Grasp barbell with shoulder-width or slightly wider grip. Lift weight to standing position. Keeping knees straight, lower bar toward top of feet by bending at the hips. After hips can no longer flex, bend waist as bar approaches top of feet. Lift bar by extending waist and hip until standing upright. Pull shoulders back slightly to avoiding rounding. Repeat.

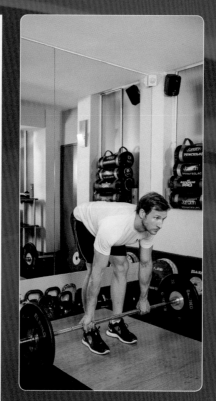
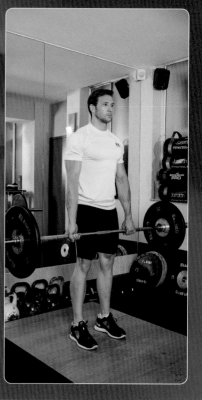

Leg extensions

▶ An isolation exercise for the quads using a specific machine. Sit in the machine. Ensure the cushioned supports are correctly placed for your body. The padding you push against should be in the ankle/lower shin area not the foot, as this would cause injuries to the ankle ligaments. Push against the pads to straighten the legs, return to start position under control.

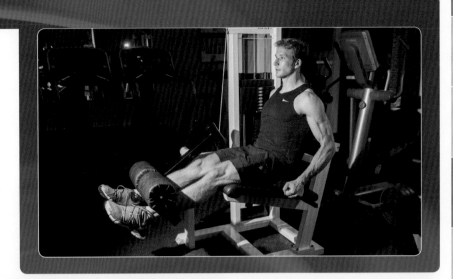

Leg curls

▶ An isolation exercise for the hamstrings using a specific machine. Sit in the machine, ensuring the supports are correctly placed for your body. The padding you push against should be at the bottom of the calf. Pull heels into backside and return to straight position under control.

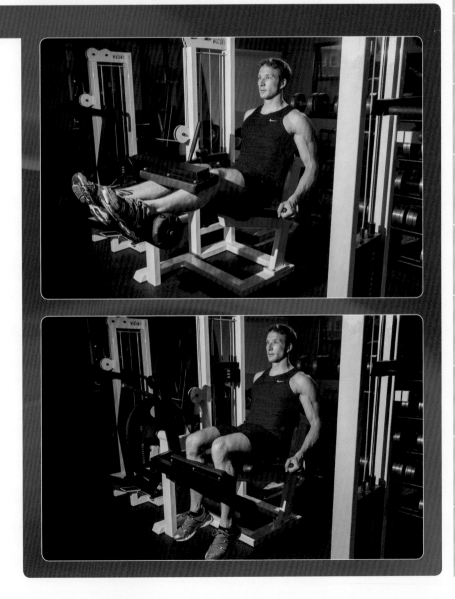

Rollouts

▶ Perform using a rollout wheel or a small barbell. Starting on the knees, with the arms straight down from the shoulders holding the handles on the wheel, allow the wheel to roll forward and in doing so stretch the whole body. Only the knees and wheel should be in contact with the ground. Return to the start position by contracting the abdominals, *ie* pull the wheel back as you return to the start position. The knees, hips and shoulders should remain in a straight line throughout the exercises. At no point should the body be bent at the hips. Repeat. It is very important to make the core/back tight when performing this exercise, as it is quite tough on the lower back at full extension.

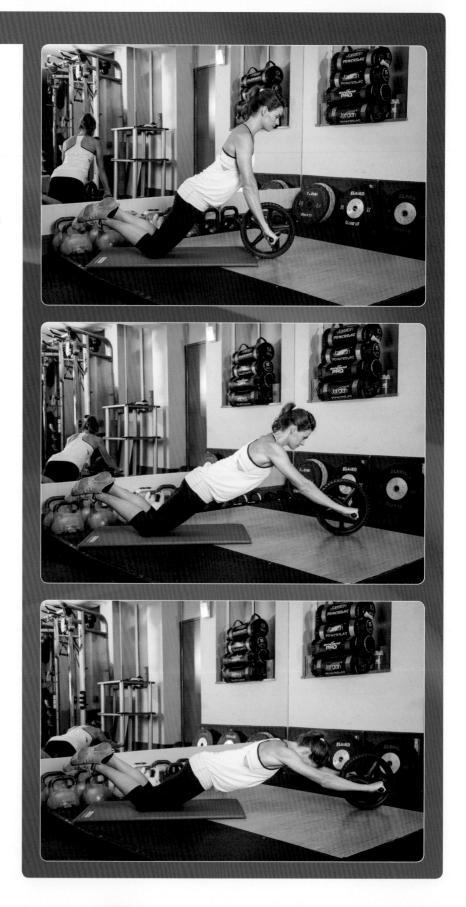

Sit-ups

▶ While lying down on the back with the legs bent, feet and knees together, sit up under control to a near vertical position so that the elbows can touch the tops of the knees. Feet should remain flat on the floor. Once vertical, lay back under control, so that the head, shoulders and elbows are back in contact with the ground. Prior to each repetition, exhale and pull the belly button in hard to contract the abdominals and hold. Repeat.

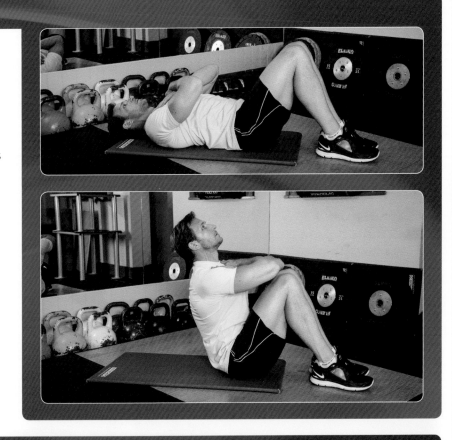

Dumbbell snatches

▶ Stand with feet apart and position a dumbbell in front, holding it with knuckles forward in a squat position with back straight. Pull dumbbell up by extending hips and knees. Jump upward extending body and shrug shoulders to pull dumbbell upward with arm, allowing elbow to pull up to side. Try to keep elbow over dumbbell as long as possible then aggressively pull body under dumbbell. Catch dumbbell at arm's length while moving into squat position. As soon as dumbbell is caught on locked-out arm in squat position, squat up into standing position with dumbbell over head. Reverse movement to lower dumbbell and repeat.

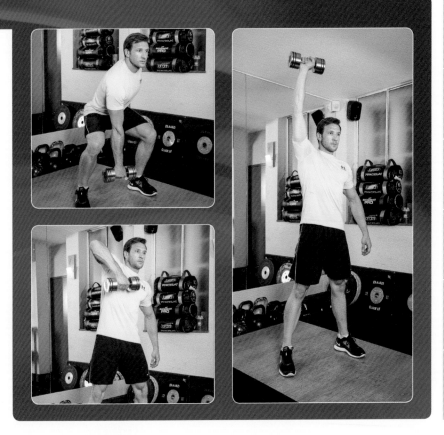

Microcycle 2
WEEK 4

Monday
Upper body
5 minutes cardio: jog, bike, row.
Mobility.
Dynamic stretch.
Try to increase weights on any exercise in which it was too easy to complete 12 last week.
Tempo 40X0.
60 seconds rest between sets.
Three sets of:
Bench press 8–12 reps.
Pull-ups to failure into inverted row 8–12 reps.
Overhead press 8–12 reps.
Incline dumbbell press 8–12 reps.
Bent-over row 8–12 reps.
Seated dumbbell shoulder press 8–12 reps.
Finisher
Power cleans 8–12 reps.

Tuesday
Legs and abs
5 minutes cardio: jog, bike, row.
Mobility.
Dynamic stretch.
Try to increase weights by 2.5–5kg from Tuesday.
Tempo 40X0.
60 seconds rest between sets.
Three sets of:
Deadlifts 8–12 reps.
Squats 8–12 reps.
Front squats 8–12 reps.
Straight-leg deadlifts 8–12 reps.
Leg extensions 8–12 reps.
Leg curls 8–12 reps.
Rollouts 8–12 reps.
Incline reverse crunch 8–12 reps.
Sit-ups 8–12 reps.
Finisher
Kettlebell swings 12–15 reps.

Wednesday
Rest.

Thursday
Upper body
5 minutes cardio: jog, bike, row.
Mobility.
Dynamic stretch.
Try to increase weights by 2.5–5kg from starting Monday.
Tempo 40X0.
60 seconds rest between sets.
Three sets of:
Bench press 6–10 reps.
Pull-ups to failure into inverted row 6–10 reps.
Overhead press 6–10 reps.
Incline dumbbell press 6–10 reps.
Bent-over row 6–10 reps.
Seated dumbbell shoulder press 6–10 reps.
Finisher
Push press 6–10 reps.

Friday
Legs and abs
5 minutes cardio: jog, bike, row.
Mobility.
Dynamic stretch.
Try to increase weights by 2.5–5kg from Tuesday.
Tempo 40X0.
60 seconds rest between sets.
Three sets of:
Deadlifts 6–10 reps.
Squats 6–10 reps.
Front squats 6–10 reps.
Straight-leg deadlifts 6–10 reps.
Leg extensions 6–10 reps.
Leg curls 6–10 reps.
Rollouts 12–15 reps.
Incline reverse crunch 12–15 reps.
Sit-ups 12–15 reps.
Finisher
TRX jump squats 20–25 reps.

Saturday
Sprint intervals.
5–10 minute jog.
Dynamic stretch.
2 x 60m sprints.
6 x 40m sprints.

Sunday
Rest.

TRX jump squats

▶ Take hold of TRX handles with your palms facing in and take a step back. Lean backward until the cables are semi-taught. Aim for your body being at about a 75 degree angle with the floor. Flex the knees and hips to squat downwards. Stand back up by explosively extending the hips and knees to jump up as high as possible in the air. Land softly and silently onto the toes and then whole foot and repeat. If you do not have access to a TRX, perform squat jumps without any apparatus.

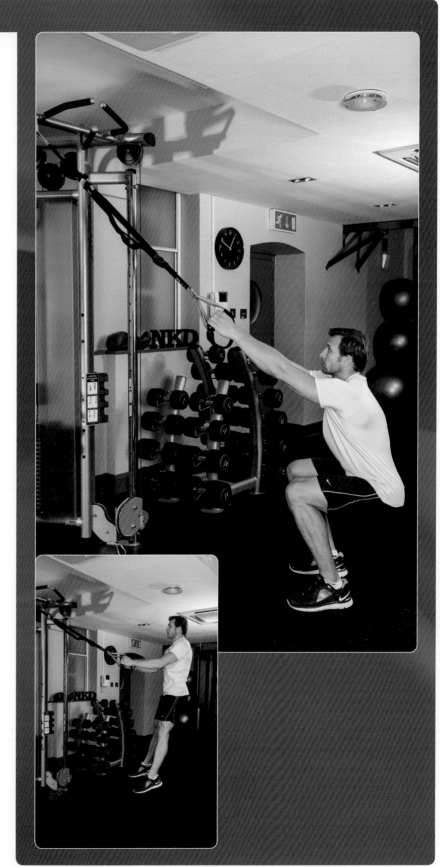

Microcycle 3
WEEK 5

Monday

Legs and abs

5 minutes cardio: jog, bike, row.
Mobility.
Dynamic stretch.
Try to choose a heavier weight than your last effort for 8–12 reps.
Tempo 3010.
60–90 seconds rest between sets.
Three sets each of:
Supersets of
1a Squats 8–12 reps.   1b Straight-leg deadlifts 8–12 reps.
2a Deadlifts 8–12 reps.   2b Front squats 8–12 reps.
3a Leg extensions 12–15 reps.   3b Leg curls 12–15 reps.
4a Weighted cable ab curls 8–12 reps.   4b Incline reverse crunch 8–12 reps.
5a Seated Olympic bar twists 8–12 reps.   5b Olympic bar side-bends 8–12 reps.
6 Farmer's walk 20m out and back.

Tuesday

Pull day.

Back and biceps

5 minutes cardio: jog, bike, row.
Mobility.
Dynamic stretch.
Try to choose a heavier weight than your last effort for 8–12 reps.
Tempo 4010
60–90 seconds rest between sets.
Three sets each of:
Supersets of
1a Chin-ups 8–12 reps.   1b Barbell curls 12–15 reps.
2a Straight-arm pull-downs 8–12 reps.   2b Inverted row 8–12 reps.
3a Pull-ups 8–12 reps.   3b Wide-grip lat pull-downs 8–12 reps.
4a Incline dumbbell hammer curls 12–15 reps.   4b Incline biceps curls 12–15 reps.
5a Close-grip pull-downs 8–12 reps.   5b Reverse grip curls 12–15 reps.
6a Biceps cable curls 12–15 reps.   6b Biceps rope hammer curls 12–15 reps.

Wednesday

Rest.

Thursday

Legs and abs

5 minutes cardio: jog, bike, row.
Mobility.
Dynamic stretch.
Try to increase weights by 2.5–5kg from Monday.
Tempo 4010.
60–90 seconds rest between sets.
Three sets each of:
Supersets of
1a Squats 8–12 reps.   1b Straight-leg deadlifts 8–12 reps.
2a Deadlifts 8–12 reps.   2b Front squats 8–12 reps.
3a Leg extensions 12–15 reps.   3b Leg curls 12–15 reps.
4a Weighted cable ab curls 8–12 reps.   4b Incline reverse crunch 8–12 reps.
5a Seated Olympic bar twists 8–12 reps.   5b Olympic bar side-bends 8–12 reps.
6 Farmer's walk 20m out and back.

Friday

Push day.

Chest, shoulders and triceps

5 minutes cardio: jog, bike, row.
Mobility.
Dynamic stretch.
Try to choose a heavier weight than your last effort for 8–12 reps.
Tempo 4010.
60–90 seconds rest between sets.
Three sets each of:
Supersets of
1a Incline dumbbell press 8–12 reps.   1b Bench press 8–12 reps.
2a Overhead press 8–12 reps.   2b Lateral raise 12–15 reps.
3a Dips 8–12 reps.   3b Wide grip bench press 8–12 reps.
4a Arnold press 8–12 reps.   4b Close-grip bench press 12–15 reps.
5a Seated dumbbell shoulder press 8–12 reps.   5b Prone incline reverse flyes 12–15 reps.
6a Standing triceps rope extension 12–15 reps.   6b Overhead triceps rope extension 12–15 reps.

Saturday
Sprint intervals.
5–10 minute jog.
Dynamic stretch.
5 x 60m sprints.
5 x 40m sprints.

Sunday
Rest.

Seated olympic bar twists

▶ Place an olympic bar across the shoulders/traps and sit on the end of a bench. Holding the bar with the hands, twist the torso around to face the wall at 90 degrees to starting position. Use the core muscles to halt the momentum the bar creates and twist back 180 degrees in the opposite direction to face the opposite wall. Twist back to the other wall and carry on repeating.

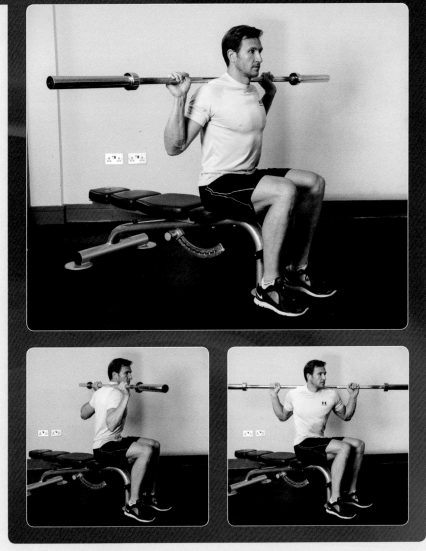

Farmer's walk

▶ Holding heavy dumbbells of equal weight in each hand carry as quickly as possible to a specific point, or round a point and back.

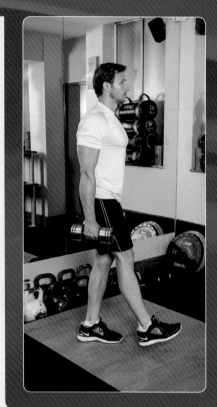
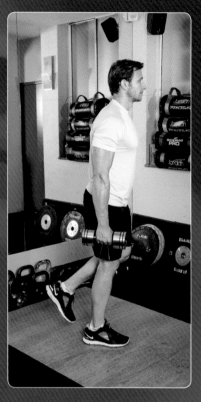

Barbell curls

▶ This exercise is performed while standing with the hands holding a barbell (palms facing away from body), which hangs down to rest on the thighs. The weight is then curled up to the shoulders. It is important to try to keep the rest of the body, especially the back, still, and to keep the elbows in at the hips. Lower dumbbell back to the start position under control and repeat.

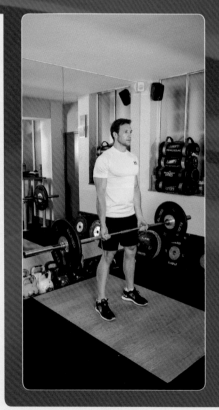
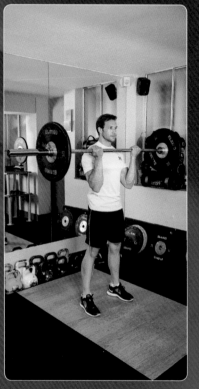

Straight-arm pull-downs

▶ Stand in front of a high pulley and grasp bar/rope attachment with arm slightly bent. Bend at the waist slightly and raise upper arms. Keeping elbows fixed, pull cable attachment down until upper arms are to sides. Return to upper position and repeat.

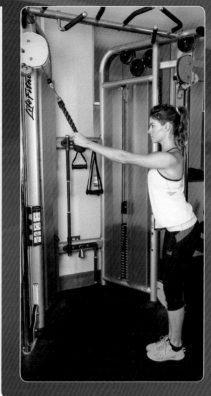
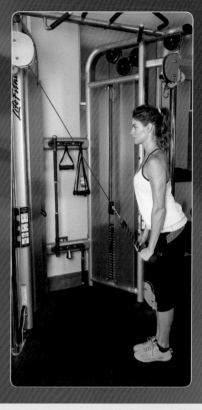

Wide-grip lat pull-downs

▶ With a wider than shoulder grip take the bar as for the pull-up and pull the bar down below the chin. Return under control to the straight arm position. Repeat.

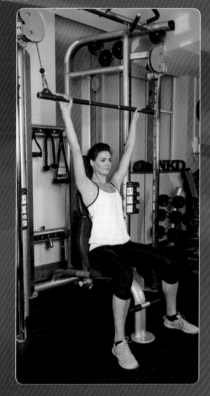
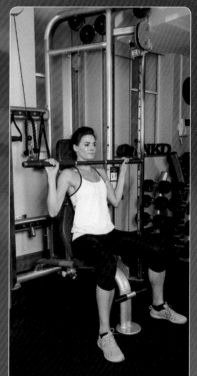

WEEK

1

2

3

4

5

6

7

8

9

10

11

12

Incline hammer curls

▶ Sit back on 45-60 degree incline bench. Let arms hang down straight holding two dumbbells with palms facing inwards. Keeping elbows to sides, raise dumbbells until forearm is vertical and palm facing shoulders. Lower to original position and repeat.

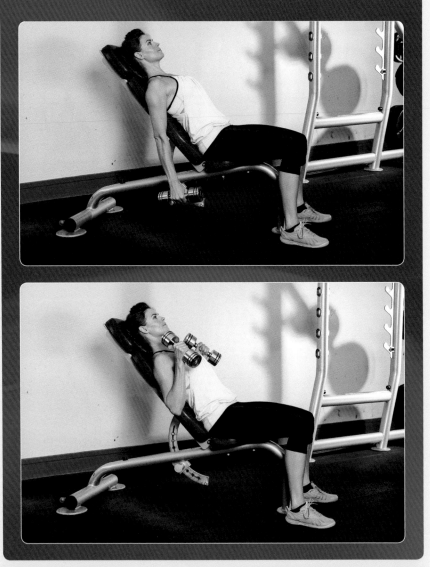

Incline biceps curl

▶ Sit back on 45-60 degree incline bench. Let arms hang down straight holding two dumbbells with palms facing forward. Keeping elbows to sides, raise dumbbells until forearm is vertical and palm facing shoulders. Lower to original position and repeat.

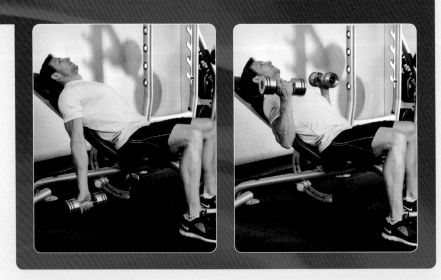

Close-grip pull-downs

▶ Grasp lat pull-down bar with a narrow grip. Pull down cable attachment to upper chest. Return until arms and shoulders are fully extended. Repeat.

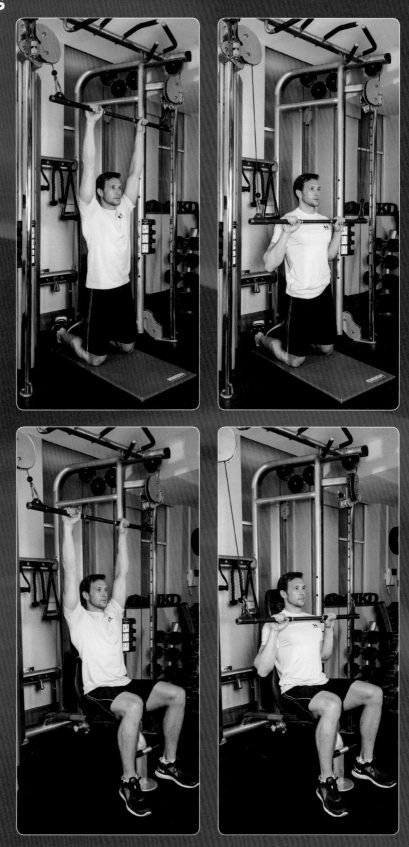

Reverse-grip curls

▶ Hold a bar with shoulder-width overhand grip, elbows to the side. Raise bar until forearms are vertical then lower under control until arms are fully extended. Repeat.

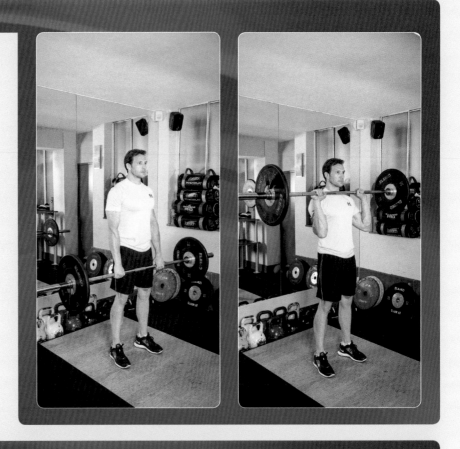

Biceps cable curls

▶ Grasp low pulley cable bar with shoulder-width underhand grip. Stand close to pulley, keep elbows locked into the side and raise bar until forearms are vertical. Lower until arms are fully extended. Repeat.

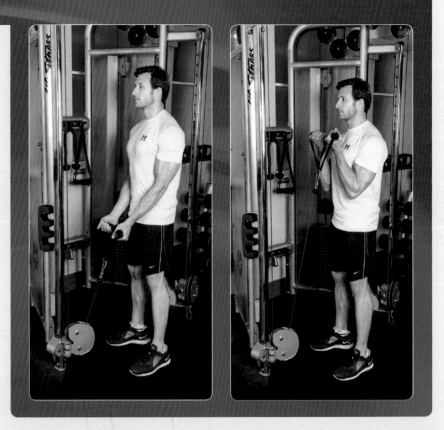

Biceps rope hammer curls

▶ Grasp cable rope with palms facing inward. Stand upright with arms straight down to sides. Keep the elbows tight into the sides, then raise the rope forward and upward with both arms until forearms are vertical. Lower until arms are fully extended. Repeat.

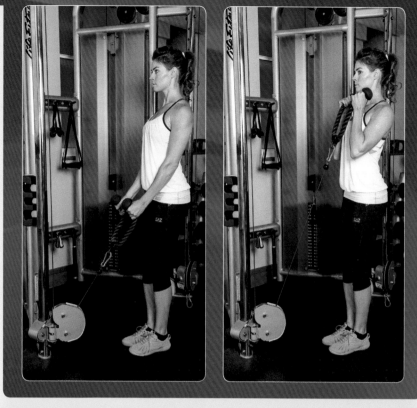

Lateral raise

▶ This exercise can be performed seated or standing. A dumbbell should be held in each hand and the arms should hang naturally down at the sides of the body. Both weights should be lifted out to the sides at the same time until at the same level as the shoulders. Then lowered under control to the start position. Repeat.

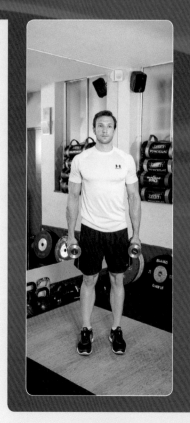

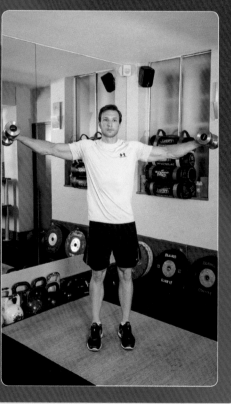

WEEK

1
2
3
4
5
6
7
8
9
10
11
12

Dips

► Place hands on parallel bars, which are shoulder-width apart. Leaning slightly forward, drop down under control until upper arms are parallel to the bars. Press up and return to start.

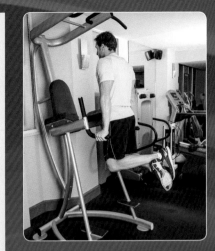
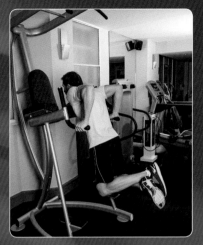

Wide grip bench press

► Lie supine on bench and take hold of barbell with a wider than shoulder-width grip. Lower weight to mid-chest. Press bar upward until arms are extended. Repeat.

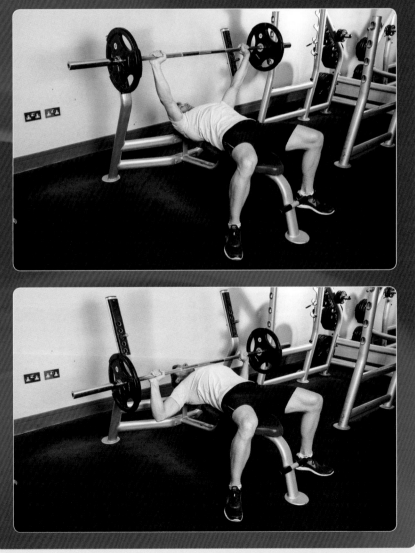

Arnold press

▶ A shoulder press with dumbbells, but the start position (weights rested on the tops of the shoulders) has the palms facing the body. As the weights are pressed they are rotated so that the palms face outwards when the weights are overhead.

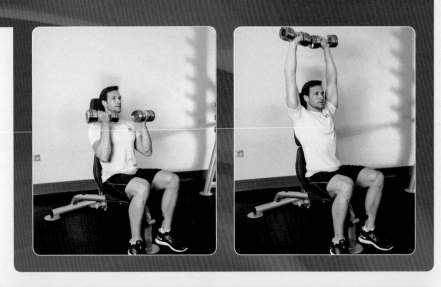

Close-grip bench press

▶ Lie on bench and grasp barbell with narrow grip. Lower weight to chest with elbows close to body. Push barbell back up until arms are straight. Repeat.

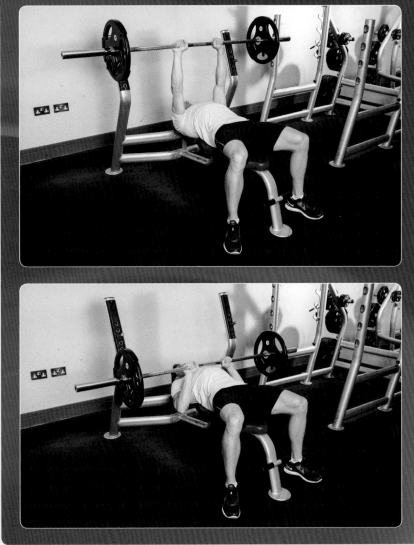

Prone incline reverse flyes

▶ Lie chest down on an incline bench. Grasp dumbbells below to each side. Raise upper arms to sides until elbows are shoulder height. Ensure fixed elbow position (10° to 30° angle) throughout exercise. Maintain height of elbows above wrists by raising little finger. Lower under control. Repeat.

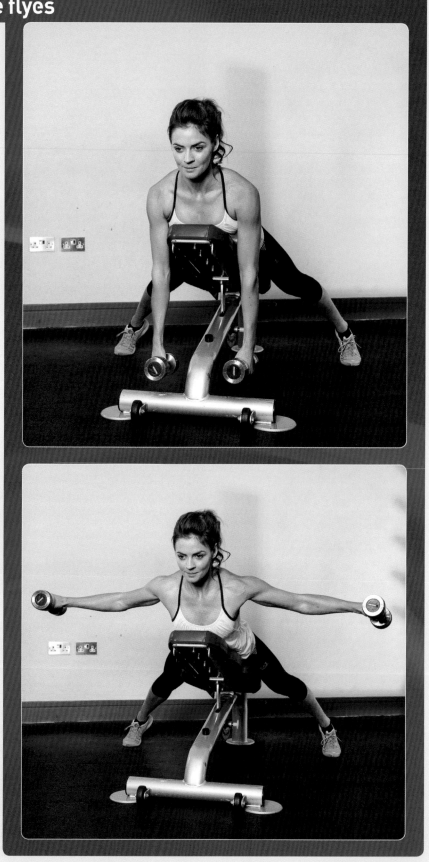

Standing triceps rope extension

▶ Stand facing a high pulley and grasp rope attachment with hands side by side (palms in), keeping the elbows positioned to the side, extend arms down. Turn palms slightly down at bottom. Return until forearm is close to upper arm and hands are in original position. Repeat.

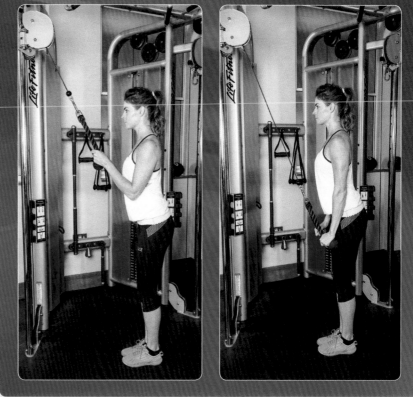

Overhead triceps rope extension

▶ Stand up straight with a strong base and position cable rope attachment behind. Ensure elbows are over head. Extend forearms over head until arms are straight. Lower under control. Repeat.

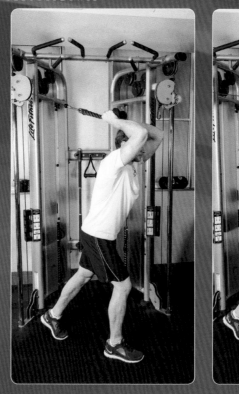
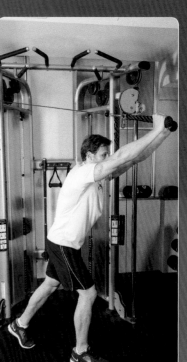

WEEK

1
2
3
4
5
6
7
8
9
10
11
12

Microcycle 3
WEEK 6

Monday
Legs and abs
5 minutes cardio: jog, bike, row.
Mobility.
Dynamic stretch.
Try to increase weights by 2.5–5kg from previous week.
Tempo 4010.
60–90 seconds rest between sets.
Three sets each of:
Supersets of
1a Squat 6–10 reps last set 2 x 10 second rest pause sets to failure.
1b Straight leg deadlifts 6–10 reps last set 2 x 10 second rest pause sets to failure.
2a Deadlifts 6–10 reps last set 2 x 10 second rest pause sets to failure.
2b Front squats 6–10 reps last set 2 x 10 seconds rest pause sets to failure.
3a Leg extensions 20–25 reps last set 2 x 10 second rest pause sets to failure.
3b Leg curls 20–25 reps last set 2 x 10 seconds rest pause sets to failure.
4a Weighted cable ab curls 6–10 reps last set 2 x 10 second rest pause sets to failure.
4b Incline reverse crunch 6–10 reps last set 2 x 10 seconds rest pause sets to failure.
5a Seated Olympic bar twists 6–10 reps.
5b Olympic bar side-bends 6–10 reps.

Tuesday
Pull day.
Back and biceps
5 minutes cardio: jog, bike, row.
Mobility.
Dynamic stretch.
Try to increase weights by 2.5–5kg from previous session of this rep range.
Tempo 4010.
60–90 seconds rest between sets.
Three sets each of:
Supersets of
1a Chin-ups 6–10 reps last set 2 x 10 seconds rest pause sets to failure.
1b Barbell curls 6–10 reps last set 2 x 10 seconds rest pause sets to failure.
2a Straight-arm pull-downs 6–10 reps last set 2 x 10 seconds rest pause sets to failure.
2b Inverted row 6–10 reps last set 2 x 10 seconds rest pause sets to failure.
3a Pull-ups 6–10 reps last set 2 x 10 seconds rest pause sets to failure.
3b Wide-grip lat pull-downs 6–10 reps last set 2 x 10 seconds rest pause sets to failure.
4a Hammer curls 6–10 reps last set 2 x 10 seconds rest pause sets to failure.
4b Incline biceps curls 6–10 reps last set 2 x 10 seconds rest pause sets to failure.
5a Close-grip pull-downs 6–10 reps last set 2 x 10 seconds rest pause sets to failure.
5b Reverse-grip curls 6–10 reps last set 2 x 10 seconds rest pause sets to failure.
6a Biceps cable curls 6–10 reps last set 2 x 10 seconds rest pause sets to failure.
6b Biceps rope hammer curls 6–10 reps last set 2 x 10 seconds rest pause sets to failure.

Wednesday

Rest.

Thursday

Legs and abs

5 minutes cardio: jog, bike, row.

Mobility.

Dynamic stretch.

Try to increase weights by 2.5–5kg from previous session of this rep range.

Tempo 4010

60–90 seconds rest between sets.

Three sets each of:

Supersets of

1a Squat 6–10 reps last set 2 x 10 seconds rest pause sets to failure.
1b Straight-leg deadlifts 6–10 reps last set 2 x 10 seconds rest pause sets to failure.

2a Deadlifts 6–10 reps last set 2 x 10 seconds rest pause sets to failure.
2b Front squats 6–10 reps last set 2 x 10 seconds rest pause sets to failure.

3a Leg extensions 20–25 reps last set 2 x 10 seconds rest pause sets to failure.
3b Leg curls 20–25 reps last set 2 x 10 seconds rest pause sets to failure.

4a Weighted cable ab curls 8–12 reps last set 2 x 10 seconds rest pause sets to failure.
4b Incline reverse crunch 8–12 reps last set 2 x 10 seconds rest pause sets to failure.

5a Seated Olympic bar twists 8–12 reps.
5b Olympic bar side-bends 8–12 reps.

Friday

Push day.

Chest, shoulders and triceps

5 minutes cardio: jog, bike, row.

Mobility.

Dynamic stretch.

Try to increase weights by 2.5–5kg from previous session of this rep range.

Tempo 4010.

60–90 seconds rest between sets.

Three sets each of:

Supersets of

1a Incline dumbbell press 6–10 reps last set 2 x 10 seconds rest pause sets to failure.
1b Bench press 6–10 reps last set 2 x 10 seconds rest pause sets to failure.

2a Overhead press 6–10 reps last set 2 x 10 seconds rest pause sets to failure.
2b Standing lateral raise 6–10 reps last set 2 x 10 seconds rest pause sets to failure.

3a Dips 6–10 reps last set 2 x 10 seconds rest pause sets to failure.
3b Wide bench press 6–10 reps last set 2 x 10 seconds rest pause sets to failure.

4a Arnold press 6–10 reps last set 2 x 10 seconds rest pause sets to failure.
4b Close-grip bench press 6–10 reps last set 2 x 10 seconds rest pause sets to failure.

5a Seated dumbbell shoulder press 6–10 reps last set 2 x 10 seconds rest pause sets to failure.
5b Prone incline reverse flyes 6–10 reps last set 2 x 10 seconds rest pause sets to failure.

6a Standing triceps rope extension 12–15 reps.
6b Overhead triceps rope extension 12–15 reps.

Saturday

Sprint intervals.

5–10 minutes jog.

Dynamic stretch.

8 x 60m sprints.

4 x 40m sprints.

Sunday

Rest.

Microcycle 3
WEEK 7

Monday
Legs and abs
5 minutes cardio: jog, bike, row.
Mobility.
Dynamic stretch.
Try to increase weights by 2.5–5kg from previous session of this rep range.
Tempo 4010.
60–90 seconds rest between sets.
Three sets each of:
Supersets of
1a Squats 5–8 reps last set 2 x 10 seconds rest pause sets to failure.   1b Straight-leg deadlifts 5–8 reps last set 2 x 10 seconds rest pause sets to failure.
2a Deadlifts 5–8 reps last set 2 x 10 seconds rest pause sets to failure.   2b Front squats 5–8 reps last set 2 x 10 seconds rest pause sets to failure.
3a Leg extensions 15–20 reps last set 2 x 10 seconds rest pause sets to failure.   3b Leg curls 15–20 reps last set 2 x 10 seconds rest pause sets to failure.
4a Weighted cable ab curls 8–12 reps last set 2 x 10 seconds rest pause sets to failure.   4b Incline reverse crunch 8–12 reps last set 2 x 10 seconds rest pause sets to failure.
5 Farmer's walk 25m out and back.

Tuesday
Pull day
Back and biceps
5 minutes cardio: jog, bike, row.
Mobility.
Dynamic stretch.
Try to increase weights by 2.5–5kg from previous session of this rep range.
Tempo 4010.
60–90 seconds rest between sets.
Three sets each of:
Supersets of
1a Chin-ups 6–10 reps last set 2 x 10 seconds rest pause sets to failure.   1b Barbell curls 15–20 reps last set 2 x 10 seconds rest pause sets to failure.
2a Straight-arm pull-downs 5–8 reps last set 2 x 10 seconds rest pause sets to failure.   2b Inverted row 5–8 reps last set 2 x 10 seconds rest pause sets to failure.
3a Pull-ups 5–8 reps last set 2 x 10 seconds rest pause sets to failure.   3b Wide-grip lat pull-downs 5–8 reps last set 2 x 10 seconds rest pause sets to failure.
4a Hammer curls 15–20 reps last set 2 x 10 seconds rest pause sets to failure.   4b Incline biceps curls 5–8 reps last set 2 x 10 seconds rest pause sets to failure.
5a Close-grip pull-downs 5–8 reps last set 2 x 10 seconds rest pause sets to failure.   5b Reverse grip curls 15–20 reps last set 2 x 10 seconds rest pause sets to failure.
6a Biceps cable curls 5–8 reps last set 2 x 10 seconds rest pause sets to failure.   6b Biceps rope hammer curls 15–20 reps last set 2 x 10 seconds rest pause sets to failure.

Wednesday

Rest.

Thursday

Legs and abs

5 minutes cardio: jog, bike, row.

Mobility.

Dynamic stretch.

Try to increase weights by 2.5–5kg from previous session of this rep range.

Tempo 4010.

60–90 seconds rest between sets.

Three sets each of:

Supersets of

1a Squats 5–8 reps last set 2 x 10 seconds rest pause sets to failure.
1b Straight-leg deadlifts 5–8 reps last set 2 x 10 seconds rest pause sets to failure.

2a Deadlifts 5–8 reps last set 2 x 10 seconds rest pause sets to failure.
2b Front squats 5–8 reps last set 2 x 10 seconds rest pause sets to failure.

3a Leg extensions 15–20 reps last set 2 x 10 seconds rest pause sets to failure.
3b Leg curls 15–20 reps last set 2 x 10 seconds rest pause sets to failure.

4a Weighted cable ab curls 8–12 reps last set 2 x 10 seconds rest pause sets to failure.
4b Incline reverse crunch 8–12 reps last set 2 x 10 seconds rest pause sets to failure.

5 Farmer's walk 25m out and back.

Friday

Push day

Chest, shoulders and triceps

5 minutes cardio: jog, bike, row.

Mobility.

Dynamic stretch.

Try to increase weights by 2.5–5kg from previous session of this rep range.

Tempo 4010.

60–90 seconds rest between sets.

Three sets each of:

Supersets of

1a Incline dumbbell press 5–8 reps last set 2 x 10 seconds rest pause sets to failure.
1b Bench press 5–8 reps last set 2 x 10 seconds rest pause sets to failure.

2a Overhead press 5–8 reps last set 2 x 10 seconds rest pause sets to failure.
2b Standing lateral raise 15–20 reps last set 2 x 10 seconds rest pause sets to failure.

3a Dips 6–10 reps last set 2 x 10 seconds rest pause sets to failure.
3b Wide bench press 5–8 reps last set 2 x 10 seconds rest pause sets to failure.

4a Arnold press 5–8 reps last set 2 x 10 seconds rest pause sets to failure.
4b Close-grip bench press 15–20 reps last set 2 x 10 seconds rest pause sets to failure.

5a Seated dumbbell shoulder press 5–8 reps last set 2 x 10 seconds rest pause sets to failure.
5b Prone incline reverse flyes 15–20 reps last set 2 x 10 seconds rest pause sets to failure.

6a Standing triceps rope extension 12–15 reps.
6b Overhead triceps rope extension 12–15 reps.

Saturday

Sprint intervals.

5–10 minute jog.

Dynamic stretch.

7 x 60m sprints.

3 x 40m sprints.

Sunday

Rest.

Microcycle 4
WEEK 8

Monday
am
15 minutes LISS.
pm
Chest and triceps
5 minutes cardio: jog, bike, row.
Mobility.
Dynamic stretch.
Use the same weight previously used for this rep range as new triset.
Tempo 4010.
60 seconds rest between sets.
Three sets each of:
Supersets of
1a Bench press 12–15 reps. 1b Bench dips 12–15 reps. 1c Kettlebell swings 15–20 reps.
2a Dumbbell press 12–15 reps. 2b Pec flyes 12–15 reps. 2c Kettlebell swings 15–20 reps.
3a Dips 12–15 reps. 3b Standing triceps rope extensions 12–15 reps. 3c Kettlebell swings 15–20 reps.
4a Incline dumbbell press 12–15 reps. 4b Incline pec flyes 12–15 reps. 4c Kettlebell swings 15–20 reps.
5a Reverse-grip incline bench press 12–15 reps. 5b EZ bar incline skull crusher 12–15 reps. 5c Kettlebell swings 15–20 reps.

Tuesday
am
15 minutes LISS and abs.
Tabata sit-ups.
pm
Legs and abs
5 minutes cardio: jog, bike, row.
Mobility.
Dynamic stretch.
Use the same weight previously used for this rep range as new triset.
Tempo 4010.
60 seconds rest between sets.
Three sets each of:
Superset of
1a Deadlifts 12–15 reps. 1b Back extensions 12–15 reps. 1c Push press 15–20 reps.
2a Back squats 12–15 reps. 2b Sissy squats 12–15 reps. 2c Push press 15–20 reps.
3a Front squats 12–15 reps. 3b Split squats (alternate leg to start) 12–15 reps. 3c Push press 15–20 reps.
4a Leg extensions 12–15 reps. 4b Leg curls 12–15 reps. 4c Push press 15–20 reps.
5 Tabata plank.

Wednesday

Rest.

Thursday

am

15 minutes LISS.

pm

Back and biceps

5 minutes cardio: jog, bike, row.

Mobility.

Dynamic stretch.

Use the same weight previously used for this rep range as new triset.

Tempo 4010.

60 seconds rest between sets.

Three sets each of:

Supersets of

1a Wide-grip pull-downs 12–15 reps.
1b Biceps barbell curls 12–15 reps.
1c Kettlebell swings 15–20 reps.

2a Close-grip chin-ups 12–15 reps.
2b Hammer curls 12–15 reps.
2c Kettlebell swings 15–20 reps.

3a Bent-over row 12–15 reps.
3b Straight-arm pull-downs 12–15 reps.
3c Kettlebell swings 15–20 reps.

4a Prone incline dumbbell row 12–15 reps.
4b Incline biceps curls 12–15 reps.
4c Kettlebell swings 15–20 reps.

5a Pull-ups to failure.
5b Inverted row 12–15.
5c Kettlebell swings 15–20 reps.

Friday

am

Rest.

pm

Legs and shoulders

5 minutes cardio: jog, bike, row.

Mobility.

Dynamic stretch.

Use the same weight previously used for this rep range as new triset.

Tempo 4010.

60 seconds rest between sets.

Three sets each of:

Supersets of

1a Plyometric box jumps 4–8 reps.
1b Dumbbell walking lunges 16–20 reps.
1c Single arm snatches on each side 8–10 reps.

2a Overhead press 12–15 reps.
2b Upright row 12–15 reps.
2c Single-arm snatches on each side 8–10 reps.

3a Front squats 12–15 reps.
3b Push press 12–15 reps.
3c Single-arm snatches on each side 8–10 reps.

4a Seated dumbbell shoulder press 12–15 reps.
4b Incline lateral raise 12–15 reps.
4c Single-arm snatches on each side 8–10 reps.

5a Back squats 12–15 reps.
5b Kettlebell goblet squats 12–15 reps.
5c Single-arm snatches on each side 8–10 reps.

6a Farmer's walk 20m.
6b Shrugs 12–15 reps.
6c Single-arm snatches on each side 8–10 reps.

Saturday

am

Intervals.

10 x 60m sprints.

Sunday

Rest.

Bench dips

► With your arms and legs straight, place your palms on the side of a bench, box or wall. Lower so that your backside moves towards the floor and your upper arms bend to become parallel to the floor. Exhale as you push up to the start point again. Repeat.

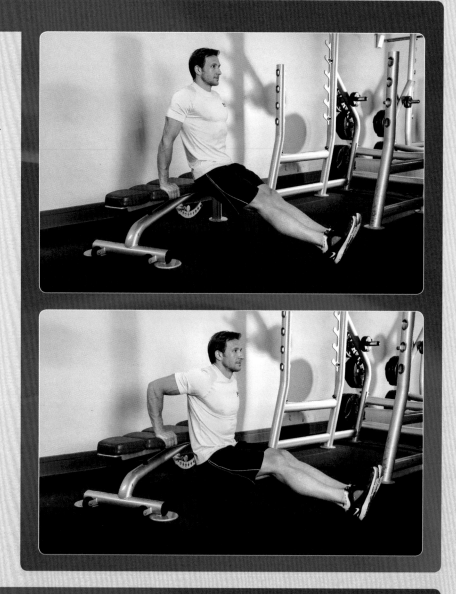

Pec flyes

► Hold two dumbbells and lie supine on bench with dumbbells above chest with arms in a slightly bent position. Internally rotate shoulders so elbows point out to sides. Lower dumbbells to sides until chest muscles are stretched with elbows fixed in same position as start. Bring dumbbells together in hugging motion until dumbbells are nearly together. Repeat.

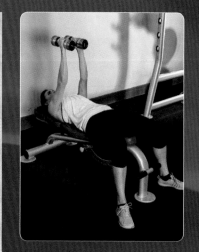
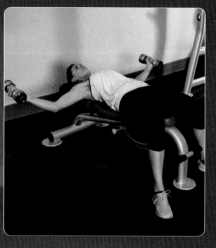

Incline pec flyes

▶ Take two dumbbells and lie supine on bench with arms straight above head fixed in slightly bent position. Bend elbows slightly and internally rotate shoulders so elbows point out to sides. Lower dumbbells outward to sides of shoulders. Keep elbows fixed in slightly bent position. When a stretch is felt in chest or shoulders, bring dumbbells back together in hugging motion above upper chest until dumbbells are nearly together. Repeat.

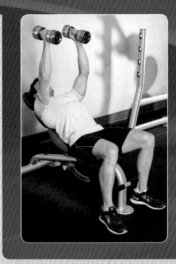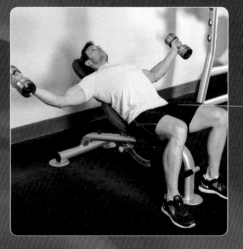

Reverse grip incline bench press

▶ Using a bench at an angle of 30 to 40 degrees lie supine on the bench with feet firmly on the floor. Grasp barbell with an underhand grip (palms facing your head). Unrack the barbell and lower to the top of your chest. Raise back to the starting position. Repeat.

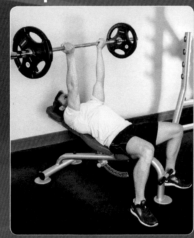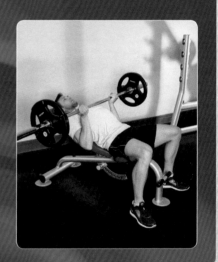

EZ bar incline skull crusher

▶ Lie on a 30 degree incline bench holding an EZ bar or barbell with narrow overhand grip. Position the barbell over shoulders with arms extended and lower to the forehead by bending elbows. Extend arms and repeat.

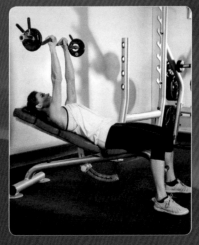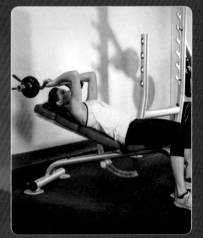

WEEK

1
2
3
4
5
6
7
8
9
10
11
12

Back extensions

► Lie prone the floor with legs out straight. Place fingers on temples. Raise torso off the floor by hyperextending the spine. Return torso to floor and repeat.

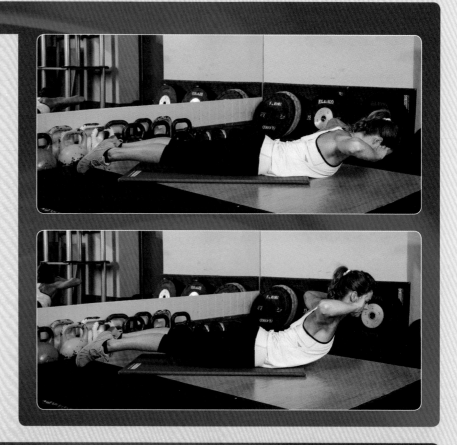

Sissy squats

► Stand with feet shoulder-width apart and grasp a fixed bar for support with one arm. Keeping hips and waist straight, bend knees to allow body to fall backwards as knees come forward. Allow heels to raise from floor. Lower body until knees are almost fully flexed or near floor. Return to original position by extending knees as heels return to floor.

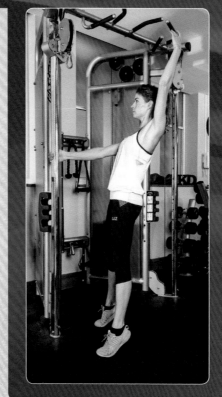
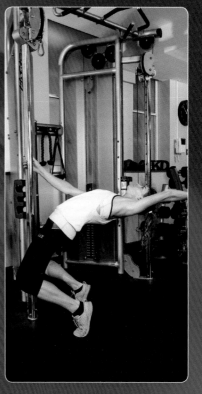

Split squat

▶ Stand with dumbbells grasped to side, one foot forward and other foot behind. Squat down by flexing knee and hip of front leg. Allow heel of rear foot to rise up while knee of rear leg bends slightly until it almost makes contact with the floor. Return to original standing position by extending hip and knee of forward leg. Repeat. Continue with opposite leg.

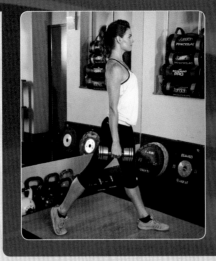 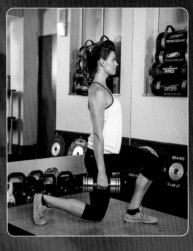

Plank

▶ Lie face down, keeping the feet and legs together, and raise the upper body by leaning on the forearms and elbows. The head should be kept up and not allowed to hang. Shoulders, hips, knees and ankles should be in line at all times; the waist/lower back particularly shouldn't be allowed to sag or be raised into the air. Once the correct position has been achieved it should be maintained for a set period.

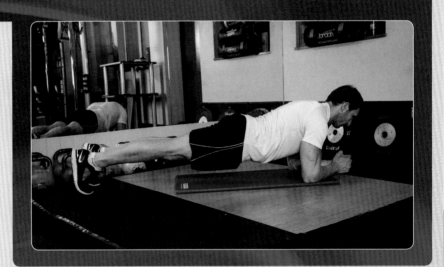

Close-grip chin-ups

▶ Grasp bar with underhand close grip. Pull body up until elbows are to sides and chin over bar. Lower body until arms and shoulders are fully extended. Repeat.

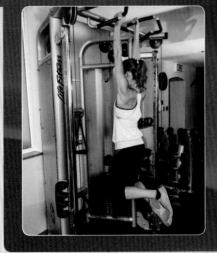 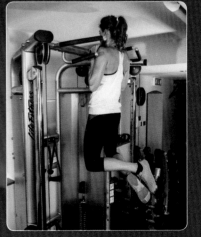

WEEK

1

2

3

4

5

6

7

8

9

10

11

12

Prone incline dumbbell row

▶ Lie prone on incline bench with chest near top of incline and with legs straddled to sides. Take a dumbbell in each hand with palms inwards. Pull dumbbells up to sides until upper arms are just beyond horizontal. Return until arms are extended and shoulder is stretched downward. Repeat.

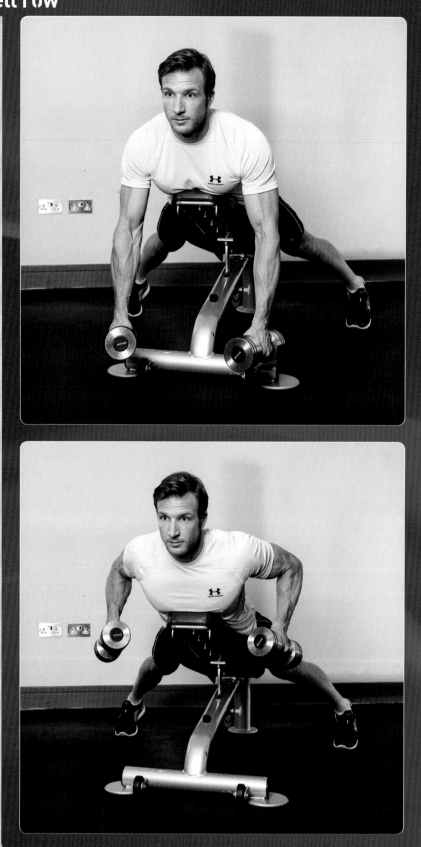

Plyometric box jumps

► With a box between one and two feet high in front of you, stand facing it with feet shoulder-width apart. Jump up on to the box from a standing start. Step down carefully and repeat.

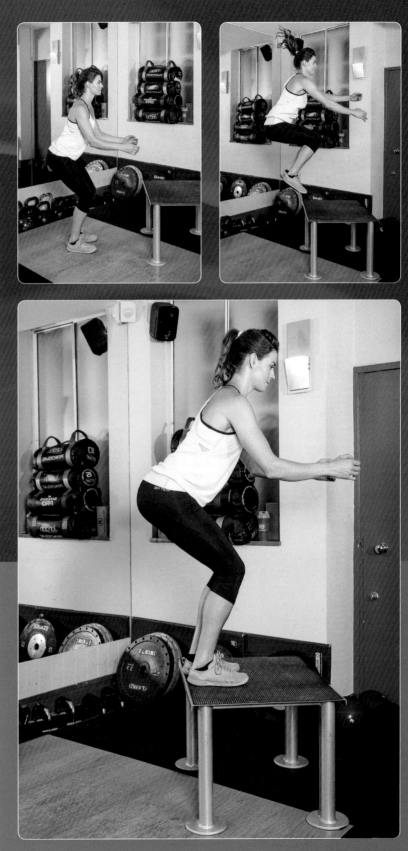

Dumbbell walking lunges

▶ Stand with dumbbells grasped to sides of the body. Step forward with first leg. Land on heel, then forefoot. Lower body by flexing knee and hip of front leg until knee of rear leg is almost in contact with floor. Stand on forward leg with assistance of rear leg. Lunge forward with opposite leg. Repeat by alternating lunge with opposite legs.

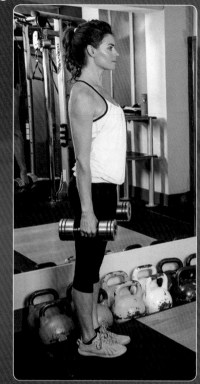
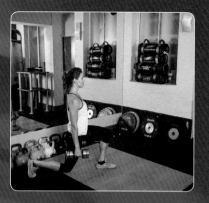
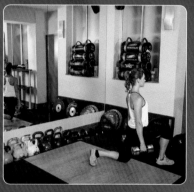

Upright row

▶ Hold a barbell at the centre. The weight is then lifted straight up to the collarbone/chin, with the elbows of both arms leading. Lower under control and repeat.

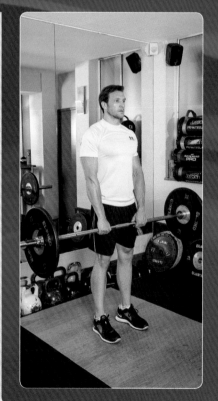
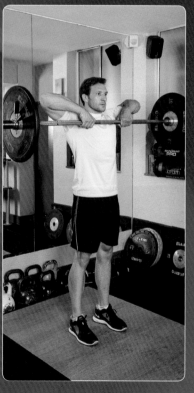

Kettlebell goblet squats

▶ Holding a kettlebell by the horns positioned close to body, stand with feet shoulder width or slightly wider apart and squat by bending the knees slightly forward while allowing hips to bend back behind, keeping back taut and knees pointed in same direction as feet. Descend until thighs are just past parallel to floor. Extend knees and hips until legs are straight. Repeat.

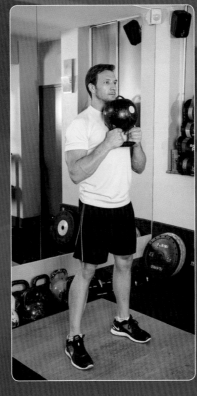
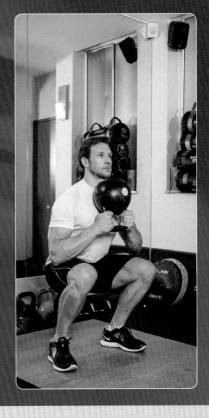

Shrugs

▶ Stand holding dumbells in the hands. Elevate shoulders as high as possible. Lower and repeat.

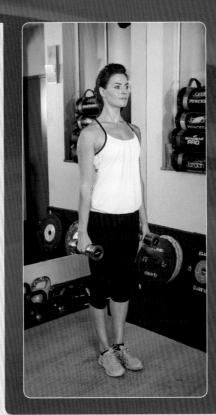
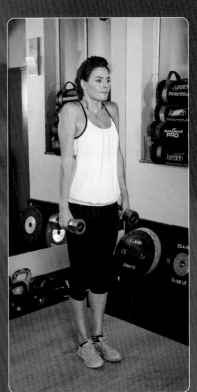

Microcycle 4
WEEK 9

Monday
am
15 minutes LISS.
pm
Chest and triceps
5 minutes cardio: jog, bike, row.
Mobility.
Dynamic stretch.
Use the same weight previously used for this rep range as new triset.
Tempo 4010.
60 seconds rest between sets.
Three sets each of:
Supersets of
1a Bench press 12–15 reps. 1b Bench dips 12–15 reps. 1c Kettlebell swings 15–20 reps.
2a Dumbbell press 12–15 reps. 2b Pec flyes 12–15 reps. 2c Kettlebell swings 15–20 reps.
3a Dips 12–15 reps. 3b Standing triceps rope extensions 12–15 reps. 3c Kettlebell swings 15–20 reps.
4a Incline dumbbell press 12–15 reps. 4b Incline pec flyes 12–15 reps. 4c Kettlebell swings 15–20 reps.
5a Reverse-grip incline bench press 12–15 reps. 5b EZ bar incline skull crusher 12–15 reps. 5c Kettlebell swings 15–20 reps.

Tuesday
am
15 minutes LISS and abs.
Tabata sit-ups.
pm
Legs and abs
5 minutes cardio: jog, bike, row.
Mobility.
Dynamic stretch.
Use the same weight previously used for this rep range as new triset.
Tempo 4010.
60 seconds rest between sets.
Three sets each of:
Superset of
1a Deadlifts 12–15 reps. 1b Back extensions 12–15 reps. 1c Push press 15–20 reps.
2a Back squats 12–15 reps. 2b Sissy squats 12–15 reps. 2c Push press 15–20 reps.
3a Front squats 12–15 reps. 3b Split squats (alternate leg to start) 12–15 reps. 3c Push press 15–20 reps.
4a Leg extensions 12–15 reps. 4b Leg curls 12–15 reps. 4c Push press 15–20 reps.
5 Tabata plank.

Wednesday
Rest.

Thursday
am
15 minutes LISS.
pm
Back and biceps
5 minutes cardio: jog, bike, row.
Mobility.
Dynamic stretch.
Use the same weight previously used for this rep range as new triset.
Tempo 4010.
60 seconds rest between sets.
Three sets each of:
Supersets of
1a Wide-grip pull-downs 12–15 reps. 1b Biceps barbell curls 12–15 reps. 1c Kettlebell swings 15–20 reps.
2a Close-grip chin-ups 12–15 reps. 2b Hammer curls 12–15 reps. 2c Kettlebell swings 15–20 reps.
3a Bent-over row 12–15 reps. 3b Straight-arm pull-downs 12–15 reps. 3c Kettlebell swings 15–20 reps.
4a Prone incline dumbbell row 12–15 reps. 4b Incline biceps curls 12–15 reps. 4c Kettlebell swings 15–20 reps.
5a Pull-ups to failure. 5b Inverted row 12–15. 5c Kettlebell swings 15–20 reps.

Friday
am
Rest.
pm
Legs and shoulders
5 minutes cardio: jog, bike, row.
Mobility.
Dynamic stretch.
Use the same weight previously used for this rep range as new triset.
Tempo 4010.
60 seconds rest between sets.
Three sets each of:
Supersets of
1a Plyometric box jumps 4–8 reps. 1b Dumbbell walking lunges 16–20 reps. 1c Single arm snatches on each side 8–10 reps.
2a Overhead press 12–15 reps. 2b Upright row 12–15 reps. 2c Single-arm snatches on each side 8–10 reps.
3a Front squats 12–15 reps. 3b Push press 12–15 reps. 3c Single-arm snatches on each side 8–10 reps.
4a Seated dumbbell shoulder press 12–15 reps. 4b Incline lateral raise 12–15 reps. 4c Single-arm snatches on each side 8–10 reps.
5a Back squats 12–15 reps. 5b Kettlebell goblet squats 12–15 reps. 5c Single-arm snatches on each side 8–10 reps.
6a Farmer's walk 20m. 6b Shrugs 12–15 reps. 6c Single-arm snatches on each side 8–10 reps.

Saturday
am
Intervals.
10 x 60m sprints.

Sunday
Rest.

Microcycle 5
WEEK 10

Monday	Tuesday
am	*am*
20 minutes LISS.	20 minutes LISS.
pm	*pm*
Shoulders and arms	***Legs and abs***
5 minutes cardio: jog, bike, row.	5 minutes cardio: jog, bike, row.
Mobility.	Mobility.
Dynamic stretch.	Dynamic stretch.
Use the same weight previously used for this rep range as new triset.	Use the same weight previously used for this rep range as new triset.
Tempo 4010.	Tempo 4010.
60 seconds rest between sets.	60 seconds rest between sets.
Four sets each of:	*Six sets each of:*
Trisets of	Supersets of
1a Overhead press 12–15 reps.	1a Deadlifts 12–15 reps.
1b Upright row 12–15 reps.	1b Incline reverse crunch 12–15 reps.
1c Front disc raise 12–15 reps.	2a Squats 12–15 reps.
Three sets each of:	2b Rollouts 12–15 reps.
Supersets of	*Three sets each of:*
2a Barbell curls 12–15 reps.	Supersets of
2b Skull crusher 12–15 reps.	3a Leg extensions 15–20 reps.
3a Prone incline reverse flyes 12–15 reps.	3b Leg curls 15–20 reps.
3b Incline lateral raise 12–15 reps.	
4a Standing triceps rope extensions 15–20 reps.	
4b Triceps overhead rope extensions 15–20 reps.	
5a Biceps cable curls 15–20 reps.	
5b Biceps rope hammer curls 15–20 reps.	

Wednesday
Rest.

Thursday
am
20 minutes LISS.
Back and biceps
5 minutes cardio: jog, bike, row.
Mobility.
Dynamic stretch.
Use the same weight previously used for this rep range as new triset.
Tempo 4010.
60 seconds rest between sets.
Three sets each of:
Supersets of
1a Chin-ups 12–15 reps. 1b Straight-arm pull-downs 15–20 reps.
2a Lat pull-downs 12–15 reps. 2b Prone incline dumbbell row 15–20 reps.
3a Single-arm row 12–15 reps. 3b Inverted row 15–20 reps.
4a Incline dumbbell hammer curls 15–20 reps. 4b Standing biceps dumbbell curls 15–20 reps.

Friday
Chest and triceps
5 minutes cardio: jog, bike, row.
Mobility.
Dynamic stretch.
Use the same weight previously used for this rep range as new triset.
Tempo 4010.
60 seconds rest between sets.
Three sets each of:
Supersets of
1a Bench press 12–15 reps. 1b Pec flyes 15–20 reps.
2a Incline dumbbell press 12–15 reps. 2b Incline pec flyes 15–20 reps.
3a Dips 12–15 reps. 3b Press-ups 15–20 reps.
4a Skull crusher 15–20 reps. 4b Close-grip bench press 15–20 reps.

Saturday
TRX jump squats.
1 minute rest between sets.
50 reps.
40 reps.
30 reps.
20 reps.
10 reps.
10 reps.
20 reps.
30 reps.
40 reps.
50 reps.

Sunday
Rest.

Front disc raise

► Grasp a weight plate disc in both hands. Position in front of upper legs with elbows slightly bent. Raise forward and upward until upper arms are above horizontal. Lower and repeat.

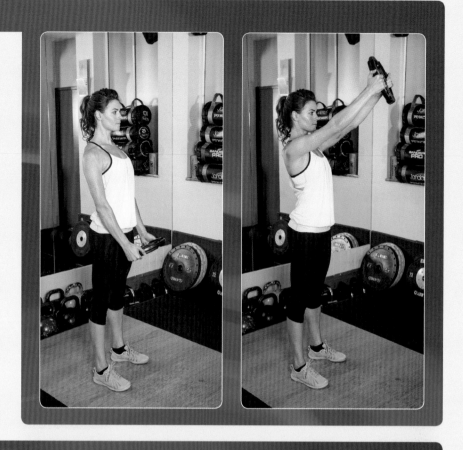

Press-ups

► Start with the hands flat, shoulder-width or very slightly more than shoulder-width apart. Ensure that your back is straight and remains straight! The legs and feet should be together throughout, bend the arms at the elbow so that the chest is about fist-height away from the floor. Once your chest is at fist-height, push down through your hands, thus straightening the arms until the elbows are straight back at the start position.

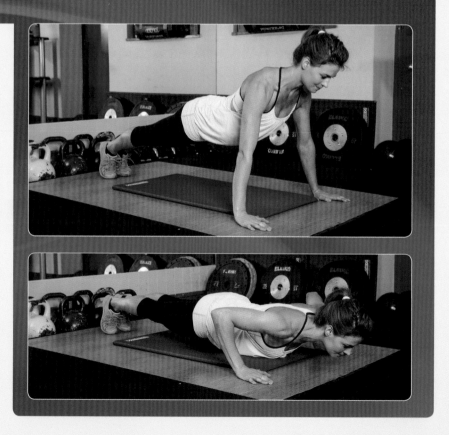

Single-arm row

▶ While resting one knee and a hand on a bench, let a dumbbell hang naturally towards the floor in the other hand. Keeping the back straight and head up, pull the weight up towards the hip and lower ribs while exhaling. Lower under control and repeat.

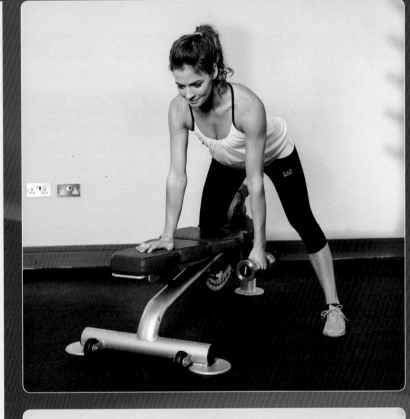

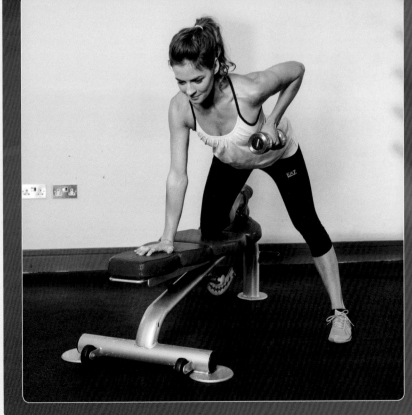

Microcycle 5
WEEK 11

Monday	
am	
25 minutes LISS.	
pm	
Shoulders and arms	
5 minutes cardio: jog, bike, row.	
Mobility.	
Dynamic stretch.	
Try to increase weights by 2.5–5kg from previous session of this rep range.	
Tempo 4010.	
90 seconds rest between sets.	
Four sets of:	
Trisets of	
1a Overhead press 8–12 reps last set 2 x 10 seconds rest/pause to failure.	
1b Upright row 8–12 reps last set 2 x 10 seconds rest/pause to failure.	
1c Front disc raise 8–12 reps last set 2 x 10 seconds rest/pause to failure.	
Three sets each of:	
Giant sets of	
2a Barbell curls 8–12 reps.	
2b Skull crusher 8–12 reps.	
2c Barbell curls to failure.	
2d Skull crusher to failure.	
3a Prone incline reverse flyes 8–12 reps.	
3b Incline lateral raise 8–12 reps.	
3c Prone incline reverse flyes to failure.	
3d Incline lateral raise to failure.	
4a Standing triceps rope extensions 8–12 reps 2 x drop sets (20–30% drop) to failure.	
4b Triceps overhead rope extensions 8–12 reps 2 x drop sets (20–30% drop) to failure.	
4c Biceps cable curls 8–12 reps 2 x drop sets (20–30% drop) to failure.	
4d Biceps rope hammer curls 8–12 reps 2 x drop sets (20–30% drop) to failure.	

Tuesday	
am	
20 minutes LISS.	
pm	
Legs and abs	
5 minutes cardio: jog, bike, row.	
Mobility.	
Dynamic stretch.	
Try to increase weights by 2.5–5kg from previous session of this rep range.	
Tempo 4010.	
60 seconds rest between sets.	
Eight sets each of:	
1a Deadlifts 8–12 reps.	
1b Incline reverse crunch 8–12 reps.	
2a Squats 8–12 reps.	
2b Rollouts 8–12 reps.	
Three sets of:	
3a Leg extensions 20–25 reps.	
3b Leg curls 20–25 reps.	

Wednesday

Rest.

Thursday

am

20 minutes LISS.

pm

Back and biceps

5 minutes cardio: jog, bike, row.

Mobility.

Dynamic stretch.

Try to increase weights by 2.5–5kg from previous session of this rep range.

Tempo 4010.

60 seconds rest between sets.

Three sets each of:

Supersets of

1a Chin-ups to failure 2 x 10 seconds rest pause sets to failure.

1b Straight-arm pull-downs 8–12 reps 2 x drop sets (20–30% drop) to failure.

2a Lat pull-downs 8–12 reps 2 x drop sets (20–30% drop) to failure.

2b Prone incline dumbbell row 8–12 reps 2 x 10 seconds rest pause sets to failure.

3a Single-arm row 8–12 reps 2 x 10 seconds rest pause sets to failure.

3b Inverted row 8–12 reps 2 x 10 seconds rest pause sets to failure.

4a Incline dumbbell hammer curls 8–12 reps 2 x 10 seconds rest pause sets to failure.

4b Standing biceps dumbbell curls 8–12 reps 2 x 10 seconds rest pause sets to failure.

Friday

Chest and triceps

5 minutes cardio: jog, bike, row.

Mobility.

Dynamic stretch.

Try to increase weights by 2.5–5kg from previous session of this rep range.

Tempo 4010.

60 seconds rest between sets.

Three sets each of:

Supersets of

1a Bench press 8–12 reps 2 x 10 seconds rest pause sets to failure.

1b Pec flyes 8–12 reps 2 x 10 seconds rest pause sets to failure.

2a Incline dumbbell press 8–12 reps 2 x 10 seconds rest pause sets to failure.

2b Incline pec flyes 8–12 reps 2 x 10 seconds rest pause sets to failure.

3a Dips 2 x 10 seconds rest pause sets to failure.

3b Press-ups to failure 2 x 10 seconds rest pause sets to failure.

4a Skull crusher 8–12 reps 2 x 10 seconds rest pause sets to failure.

4b Close-grip bench press 8–12 reps 2 x 10 seconds rest pause sets to failure.

Saturday

Supersets of

1a TRX jumps squats.

1b Walking lunges (no weight).

1 minute rest between sets.

50 reps of each.

40 reps of each.

30 reps of each.

20 reps of each.

10 reps of each.

10 reps of each.

20 reps of each.

30 reps of each.

40 reps of each.

50 reps of each.

Sunday

Rest.

Microcycle 5
WEEK 12

Monday
am
25 minutes LISS.
Abs
Sit-ups 10 reps three sets 30 seconds rest between.
Abs rollouts 10 reps three sets 30 seconds rest between.
Lying leg raises 10 reps three sets 30 seconds rest between.
pm
Chest and back
5 minutes cardio: jog, bike, row.
Mobility.
Dynamic stretch.
Try to use same weights from previous session of this rep range.
Tempo 4010.
60 seconds rest between sets.
10 sets each of 8–12 reps:
1a Dips. 1b Chin-ups.
2a Inverted row. 2b Dumbbell press.

Tuesday
am
25 minutes LISS.
Abs
Sit-ups 10 reps three sets 30 seconds rest between.
Rollouts 10 reps three sets 30 seconds rest between.
Incline reverse crunch 10 reps three sets 30 seconds rest between.
pm
Legs
5 minutes cardio: jog, bike, row.
Mobility.
Dynamic stretch.
90 seconds rest between sets.
1 complex set, 3 rotations same barbell weight throughout.
Front squats 8–12 reps.
Barbell lunges 20–24 reps.
Back squats 8–12 reps.
Jump squats to failure.
2 complex sets, 3 rotations same dumbbells in hands throughout.
Step-ups 8–12 reps each leg.
Side step-ups 8–12 reps each leg.
Walking lunges 20–24 reps.
Split squats 8–12 reps each leg.

Wednesday
Rest.

Thursday

am

20–25 minutes LISS.

Abs

Sit-ups 10 reps three sets 30 seconds rest between.

Abs rollouts 10 reps three sets 30 seconds rest between.

Lying leg raises 10 reps three sets 30 seconds rest between.

pm

5 minutes cardio: jog, bike, row.

Mobility.

Dynamic stretch.

Try to use same weights from previous session of this rep range.

Tempo 4010.

90 seconds rest between sets.

Shoulders and arms

Three sets each of:

Giant sets of

1a Seated dumbbell shoulder press 8–12 reps.
1b Upright row 8–12 reps.
1c Incline lateral raise 8–12 reps.
1d Prone incline reverse flyes 8–12 reps.
1e Seated dumbbell shoulder press (same weight as 1a, to failure).

2a Close-grip chin-ups to failure.
2b Barbell curls 8–12 reps.
2c Standing hammer curls 8–12 reps.
2d Incline curls 8–12 reps.
2e Barbell curls (same weight as 2b, to failure).

3a Dips 8–12 reps.
3b Close-grip bench press 8–12 reps.
3c Triceps dumbbell extensions 8–12 reps.
3d Bench dips 8–12 reps.
3e Dips to failure.

Friday

am

20–25 minutes LISS.

Abs

Sit-ups 10 reps three sets 30 seconds rest between.

Rollouts 10 reps three sets 30 seconds rest between.

Incline reverse crunch 10 reps three sets 30 seconds rest between.

pm

Legs

5 minutes cardio: jog, bike, row.

Mobility.

Dynamic stretch.

Try to use same weights from previous session of this rep range.

Tempo 4010.

60 seconds rest between sets.

1 Squats 10 sets 10 reps 1 minute rest between.

2 Deadlifts 10 sets 10 reps 1 minute rest between.

3 Leg extensions 12–15 reps, 2 x rest/pause sets for last set.

4 Leg curl 12–15 reps, 2 x rest/pause sets for last set.

Saturday

am

Rest.

pm

Chest and back

5 minutes cardio: jog, bike, row.

Mobility.

Dynamic stretch.

Try to use same weights from previous session of this rep range.

Tempo 4010.

60 seconds rest between sets.

1 Incline dumbbell press 10 sets 10 reps 1 minute rest between.

2 Pull-ups 10 sets 10 reps 1 minute rest between.

3 Pec flyes 3 sets 12–15 reps, 2 x rest/pause sets for last set.

4 Straight-arm pull-down 3 sets 12–15 reps, 2 x rest/pause sets for last set.

Sunday

Rest.

Jump squats

▶ From a standing position with feet shoulder-width apart and parallel to eachother, lower down into a squat. Once at the bottom, jump up and explode into the air by extending the hips and knees powerfully. Land softly (and where possible silently) into a squat again, first onto the toes and then onto the heel to repeat.

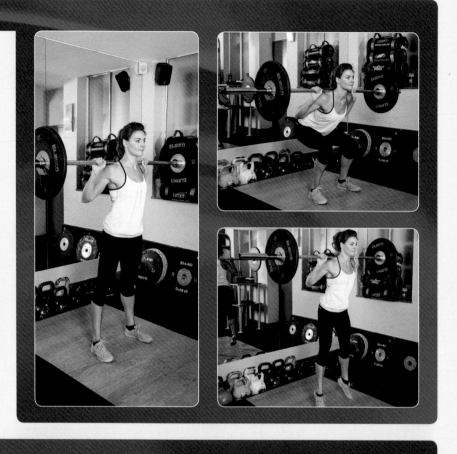

Step-ups

▶ With a step (around a foot high) in front of you, step up with the right foot, then the left foot, down with the right foot and down with the left foot. Always ensure the whole foot, not just half, is placed on the step. It's important to changes the lead step foot so they share the initial (harder) step-up equally – eg perform ten right foot first, then ten left foot first.

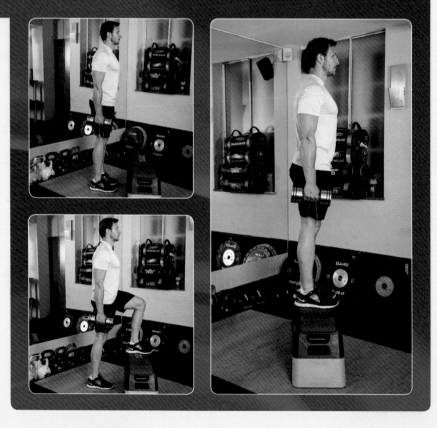

Side step-ups

▶ Stand side on to a bench. Lift leg and place foot on bench to side slightly forward of straight knee. Stand on bench by straightening leg and pushing body upward. Step down returning feet to original position. Repeat.

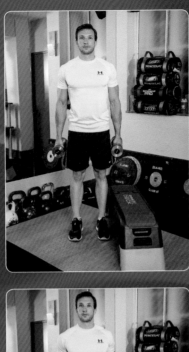

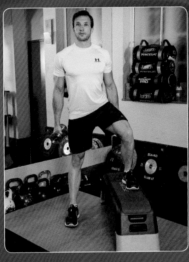

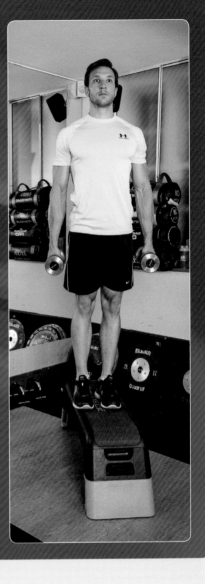

Tips for success

1. Stick to the exercises, reps, sets, tempo and timings given.
2. Keep every session intense. Take it easy and it doesn't work.
3. Imagine the BBC documentary cameras are on you the whole time and the world is watching. Train as if they are.
4. Drink 1–1.5 litres of water each session.
5. Fill in your training diary.
6. Get your nutrition and supplements right.

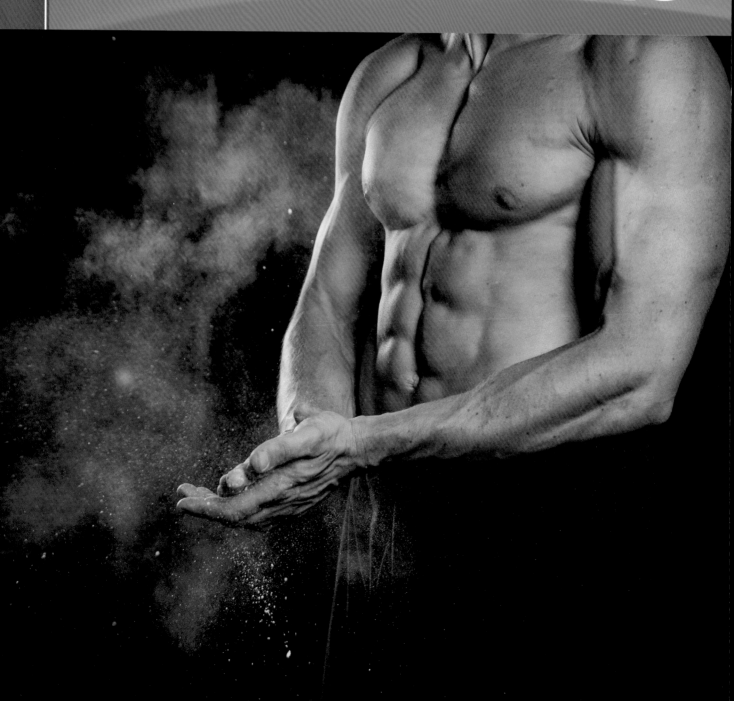

CHAPTER 7
REGRESSIONS & PROGRESSIONS

The previous chapter outlined the programme you should aim to follow for the next 12 weeks, which combined with a sensible nutrition plan and good rest, should see you obtain that figure/physique you've always wanted. However, some of you will be unable to complete a chin-up, others will find press-ups too easy and some may find their gym doesn't have a piece of equipment. What then? This chapter gives you some alternative exercises, so whoever you are and wherever you are, you can make it work for you.

The following pages show various exercises that can be used to replace some of the exercises in the training programme in the previous chapter. For those exercises which are regressions or progressions of specific exercises from the programme, this has been noted next to the exercise description. For example, if you find dips too hard, we have band supported dips, where a large elastic band is used to take some of your body weight and enable you to complete the exercise for the desired rep range in the programme. Equally, for some of you, doing 6–8 dips may be really easy, in which case, weighted dips can be used to make the exercise that little bit harder and thus help you reach failure within the rep range with the desired tempo. Remember, it's all about creating intensity in the workout, however, this needs to happen under the guidelines of the training. If the exercise is too hard and you can't complete it at all, there is no intensity whatsoever. We want you to fail, but you need to fail at 8-12 reps, not 1-2! Therefore, use the regressions to ensure your body is pushed, you feel it working and it is forced to adapt. Equally, if the exercise is too easy and you can complete the desired reps without breaking a sweat, you may as well be watching the TV with your feet up! Look at the progression and make things hard on yourself (within the prescribed rep ranges). You'll thank me in the long run, even if you are cursing me at the time.

Other exercises have been included that can either be used to replace exercises in the programme in the previous chapter or are exercises from one of the 'What Next' continuation programmes in the closing stages of this book. For most of you, you won't need to utilise these exercises until you come to try these other programmes, however, some of you will find, for example, that you don't have access to an abs wheel so you can't do 'rollouts' and therefore have to use 'hand walk-outs'. Others may get a lower limb injury (pulled hamstring, painful knee etc) while doing this programme. Unfortunately injuries happen – we just have to accept it and try our best to succeed and repair. Those that do

suffer a lower limb injury may have to utilise kneeling triceps rope extension instead of the standing variety. Or lastly, your gym may not have a barbell for bench press, in which case you'll have to use dumbbell press instead.

The following list is far from exhaustive – there are hundreds of exercises out there. If you are forced to adapt the training programme due to unavailability of kit or injury, try to substitute exercises that exercise the same muscles in the same way, i.e. chest exercise for chest exercise, compound exercise for compound where the injury will allow. Finally, if you can't find something suitable in the following pages, use the internet, YouTube and websites such as Men's Health to look for videos and alternative exercises.

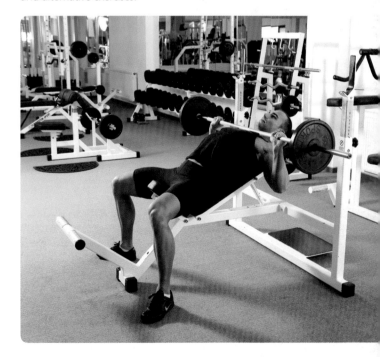

Band-assisted pull-ups

Regression of pull-up
▶ Step up and grasp the bar with an overhand grip. Kneel into the band and lower the body down with arms extended. Pull body up until chin reaches height of hands. Lower body until arms and shoulders are fully extended. Repeat.

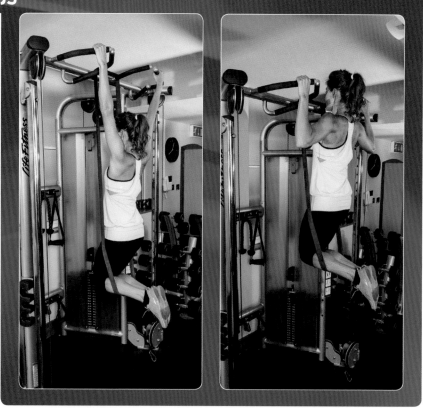

Band press-ups

Progression of press-ups
▶ Take the band behind your back and place your hands in the ends of the bands so that the band is in the palm of the hands. Kneel down and get into the press-up position. Perform press-ups as normal, in a controlled manner against the elasticity of the band.

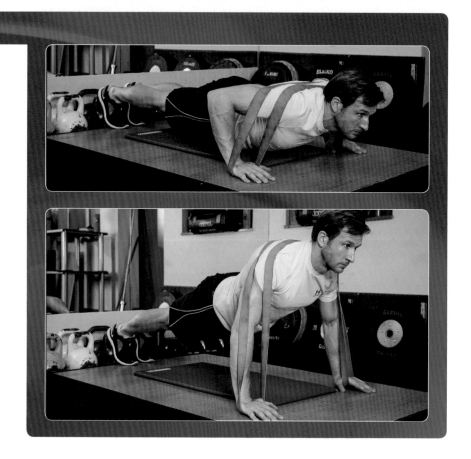

Band-supported dip

Regression of dip

▶ Step up and grasp the dip bars. Kneel or stand into the band and lower the body down with arms bent. Push the body up until the arms are straight. Lower the body until elbows are bent to 90 degrees. Repeat.

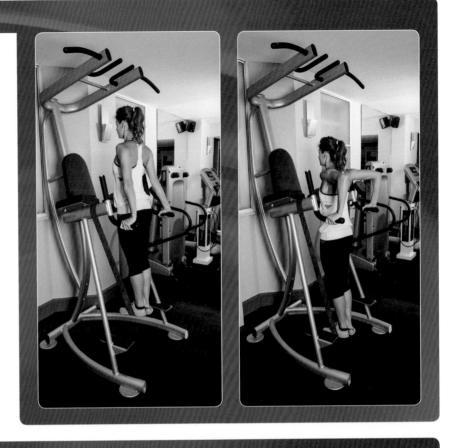

Barbell lunge

▶ Place the bar across the shoulders and grasp barbell to sides. Lunge forward with first leg. Land on heel, then forefoot. Lower body by flexing knee and hip of front leg until knee of rear leg is almost in contact with floor. Return to original standing position by forcibly extending hip and knee of forward leg. Repeat by alternating lunge with opposite leg.

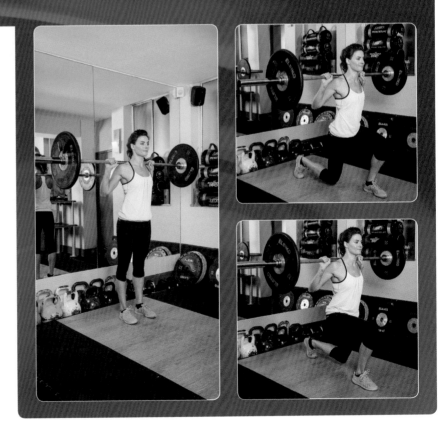

Bent-over reverse flyes

Alternate of Prone Incline reverse flyes

► Bend over. Hold dumbbells with each hand with a slight bend in the elbows and palms facing each other. Raise upper arms to sides until elbows are shoulder height. Maintain upper arms perpendicular to torso and fixed elbow position (10° to 30° angle) throughout exercise. Maintain elbows height above wrists by raising little finger side uppermost. Lower and repeat..

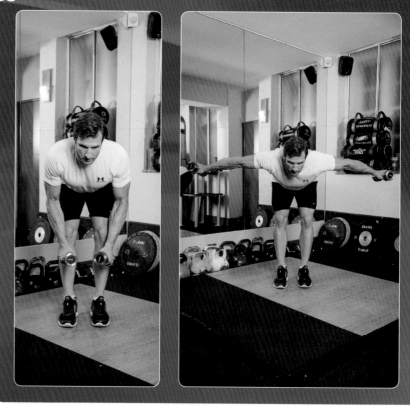

Bodyweight lunge

Regression of lunge exercises

► Stand with hands on hips, by sides or across chest. Lunge forward with first leg. Land on heel, then forefoot. Lower body by flexing knee and hip of front leg until knee of rear leg is almost in contact with the floor. Return to original standing position by forcibly extending hip and knee of forward leg. Repeat by alternating lunge with opposite leg.

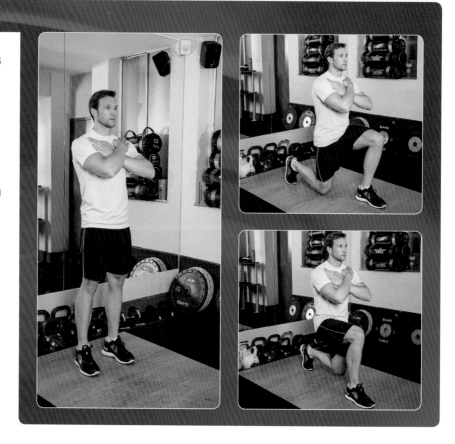

Bodyweight squat

Regression of squat exercises

▶ Stand with arms by the sides, in front or folded across the chest. Squat down by bending hips back while allowing knees to bend forward, keeping back straight and knees pointed in same direction as feet. Descend until thighs are just past parallel to floor. Squat up by extending knees and hips until legs are straight. Return and repeat.

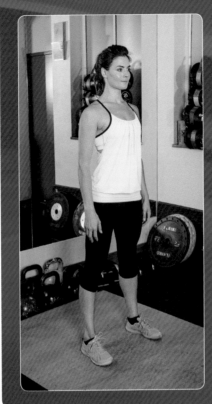
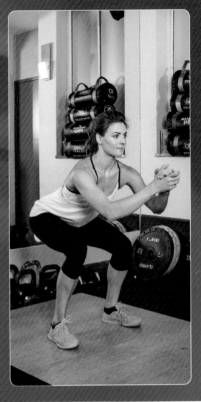

Bradford press

▶ Press a barbell so that it is over your head, but don't lock the elbows. Lower the barbell behind your head, then press back up and back to the front of the body. This would constitute one rep.

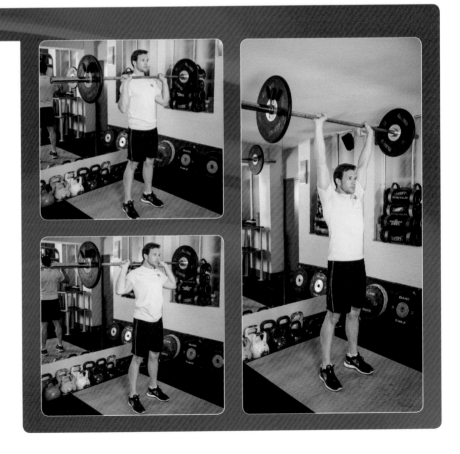

Cable crossover

▶ Grasp two opposing high pulley handles attached to high pulleys to each side. Bend over slightly by flexing hips and knees. Bend elbows slightly and internally rotate shoulders so elbows are back initially. Bring cable attachments together in hugging motion with elbows in fixed position. Keep shoulders internally rotated so elbows are pointed upward at top and out to sides at bottom. Return to starting position until chest muscles are stretched. Repeat.

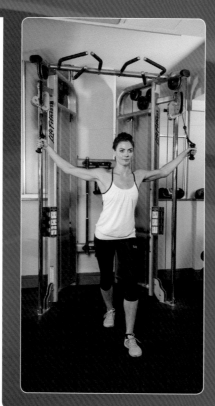 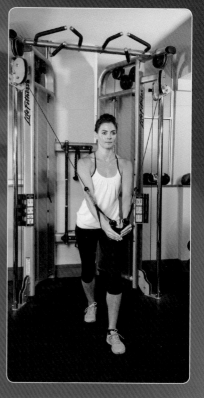

Dumbbell press

Alternate of bench press

▶ Very similar to the bench press, but instead of a bar (barbell) two dumbbells constitute the weight to be moved. Perform in a very similar way to the bench press, keeping elbows at a 45 degree angle to body, lower weights to chest and push back up to start position.

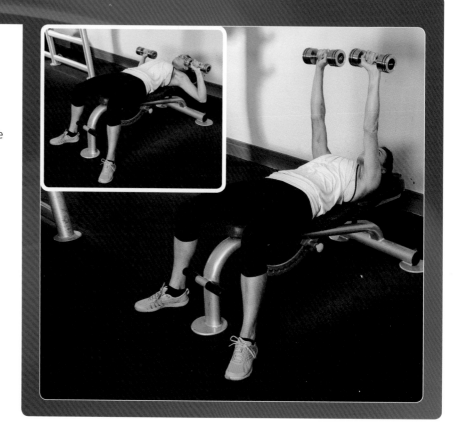

Dumbbell zottman curls

▶ Stand holding a pair of dumbbells at your sides with a palms-up (supinated) grip. Keeping your elbows pinned to your sides, simultaneously curl both dumbbells toward your shoulders. At the top, pause and squeeze your biceps hard, then rotate the weights until your palms are in the forward (pronated) position. Keeping your hands in this position, slowly lower the dumbbells toward your thighs, stopping short of lockout. Pause and turn your palms back to the supinated starting position. Repeat.

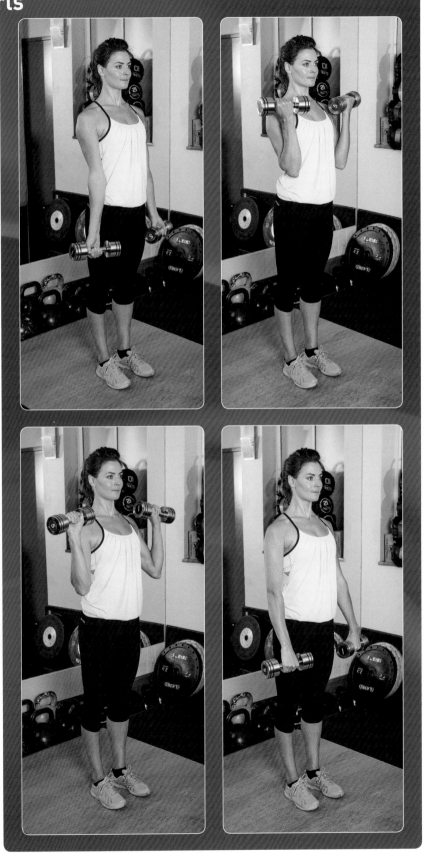

Hand walk-out

Regression of rollout

▶ From a kneeling position place the palms onto the floor. Shift the weight from the feet onto the hands and begin walking one hand forward. Walk the hands out until in a press-up position with a straight back. Walk back to the upright position and repeat. Can be performed from standing as well.

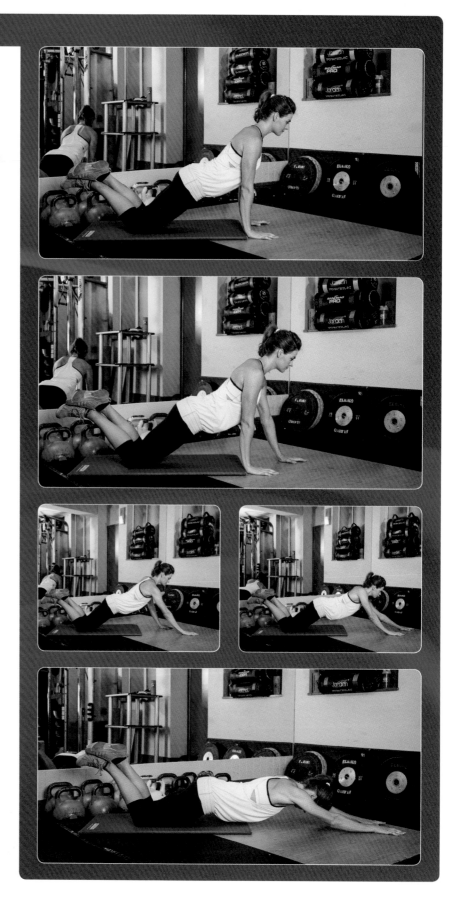

Incline lateral raise

▶ Seated on a 60 degree incline bench holding dumbells in the hands, let the arms hang naturally at the sides. Raise the arms up to the sides until level with the shoulders. Lower under control and repeat.

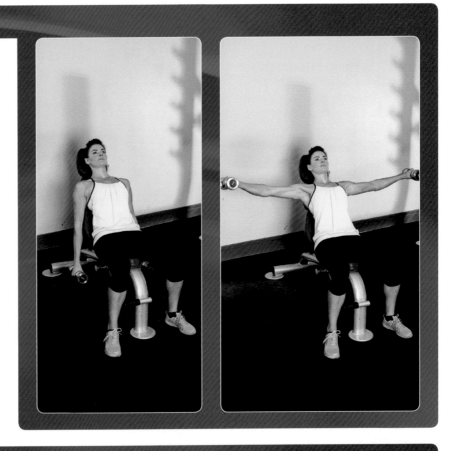

Kneeling triceps rope extension

Alternate of standing triceps rope extension

▶ Kneel down in front of a high pulley and grasp rope attachment with clinched hands side by side (palms in). Position elbows to side and extend the arms down. Turn palms slightly down at bottom. Return until forearm is close to upper arm and hands are in original position. Repeat.

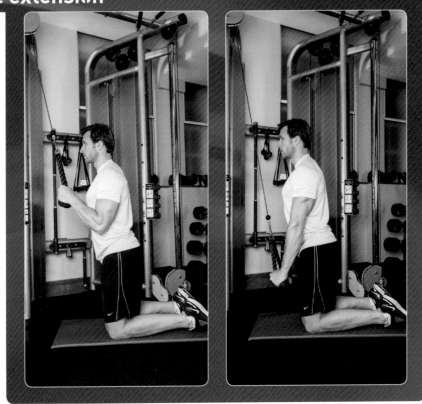

Low cable crossover

► Set two pulley handle attachments at the lowest point and stand with pulleys to each side. Bend elbows slightly so elbows are back initially. Bring cable attachments together in hugging motion with elbows in fixed position. Return to starting position until chest muscles are stretched. Repeat.

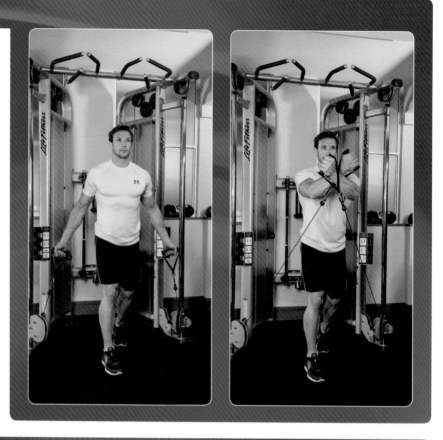

Military press

Alternate of shoulder press

► While standing straight, holding a barbell across the chest, tuck the pelvis under by holding the abs tight. As you exhale, push the weight upwards, allowing the head to come through the arms to ensure the weight goes above the shoulders and not in front of them. Lower under control. Repeat. Standing makes your core work far more, but you must ensure you don't lean back to use your stronger chest muscles.

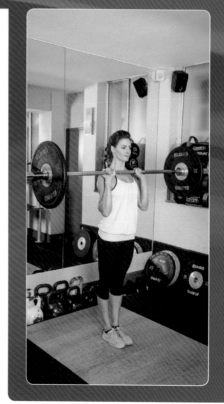

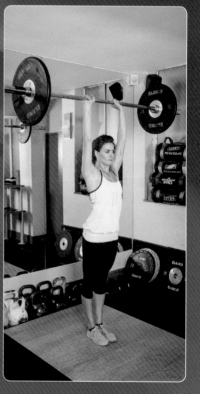

Seated cable row

► Sit on a bench with a straight back and grasp cable attachment. Place feet on vertical platform/position them to give support. Ensure slight bend in knees. Pull cable attachment to waist, keeping lower back straight. Keep shoulders back and push chest forward while arching back to ensure correct form. Return until arms are extended. Repeat.

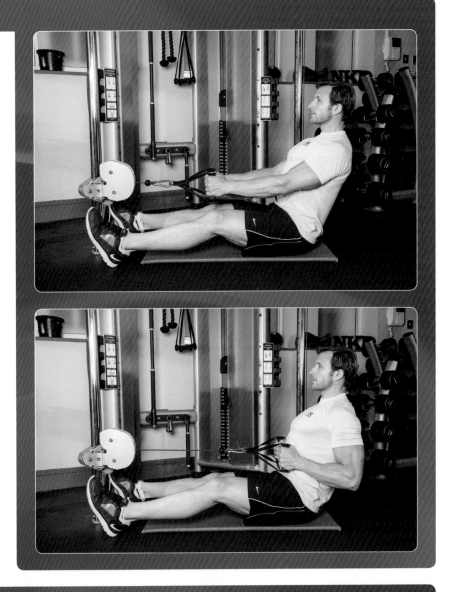

Seated dumbbell calf raise

► While sat on the edge of a bench, a dumbbell is placed on the fleshy part of the end of the quad/knee of the leg to be exercised and the weight is 'lifted' by going on to tiptoe with the feet. Return to the start point. Repeat.

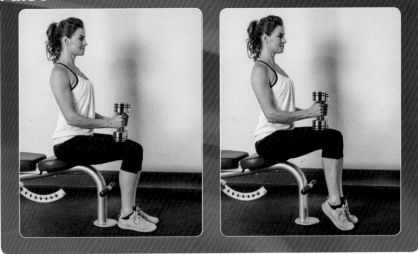

Side plank

▶ Lie on side and place forearm on mat under shoulder perpendicular to body. Place upper leg directly on top of lower leg and ensure straight knees and hips. Raise body upward by straightening waist so body is ridged. Hold position with knees, hips and shoulders in line. Repeat with opposite side.

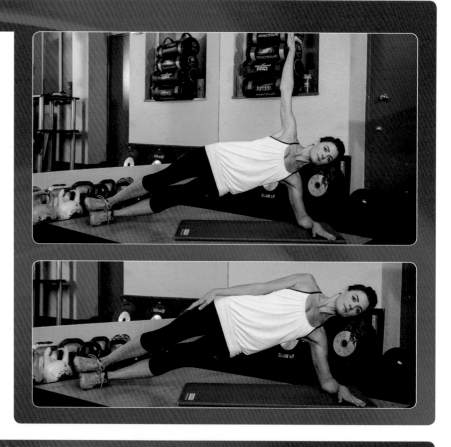

Standing biceps dumbbell curls

▶ Hold two dumbbells to sides, palms facing out, arms straight. Keeping elbows into the sides, raise dumbbells until forearm is vertical and palm faces shoulder. Lower to original position and repeat.

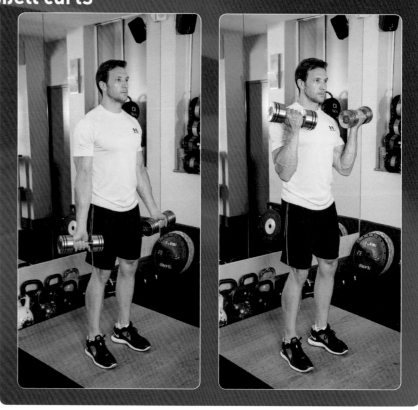

Standing calf raise

▶ Place a barbell on the shoulders standing either on the floor, or on the edge of a step. Raise up on to tiptoe from a position with the feet pointing forwards just under shoulder-width apart. Slowly return to the start point.

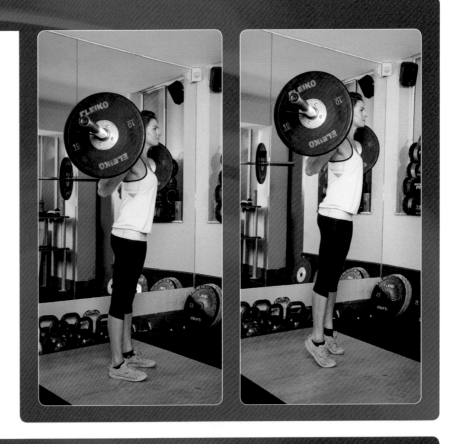

Standing dumbbell shoulder press

▶ Hold two dumbbells on the top of the shoulders with a slightly wider than shoulder-width overhand grip. Press dumbbells upward until arms are extended overhead. Lower and repeat.

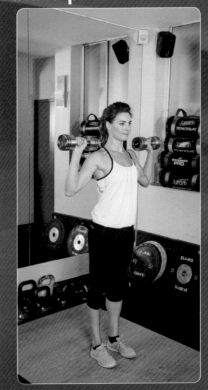
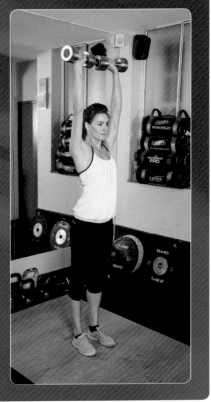

Standing hammer curls

► Hold two dumbbells to sides, palms facing in, arms straight. Keeping elbows into the sides, raise dumbbells until forearm is vertical keeping palms facing inwards. Lower to original position and repeat.

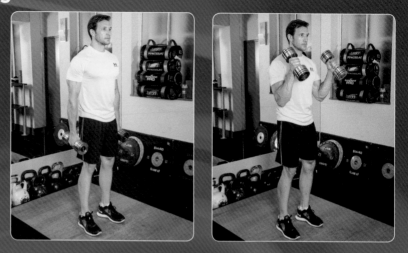

Triceps dumbbell extension

► While lying flat on a bench, hold a dumbbell in each hand straight above the head. Inhale as you bend the elbows, still keeping your upper arms at right angles to the floor. The lower arms then move so they're parallel with the ground. Return to the start position. Repeat.

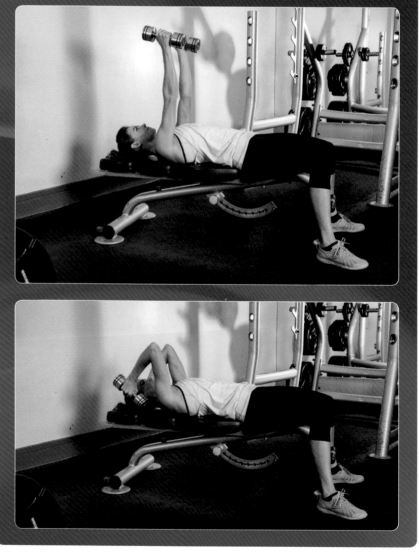

Triceps kickback

▶ Bend over and grasp dumbbells and position upper arms parallel to floor. Extend arms until it is straight. Return to start position and repeat.

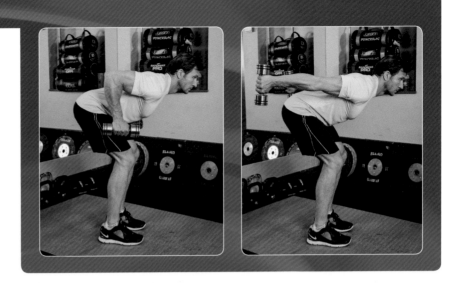

Triceps skull crusher

▶ Lie on a flat bench holding an EZ bar or barbell with narrow overhand grip. Position the barbell over shoulders with arms extended and lower to the forehead by bending elbows. Extend arms and repeat.

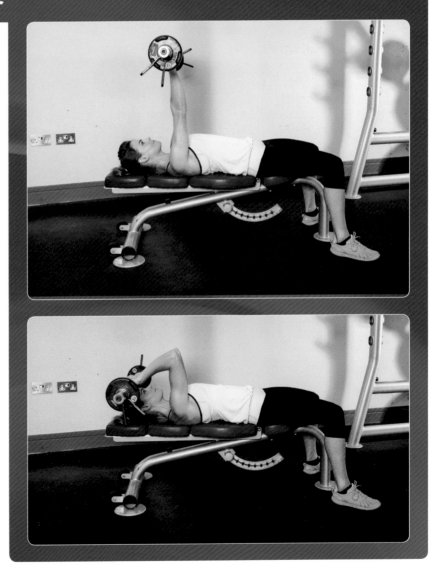

Underhand grip lat pull-down

► This exercise can be carried out kneeling or seated. Take hold of a lat pull-down bar with a close grip. Pull down cable attachment to upper chest. Return until arms and shoulders are fully extended. Repeat.

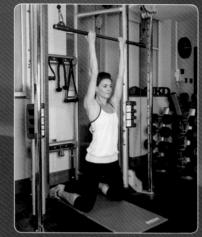
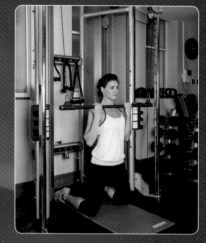

Weighted pull-up

Progression of pull-up
► Place weight on belt around waist or place dumbbell between lower legs. Step up and grasp bar with overhand wide grip. Pull body up until chin is above bar. Lower body until arms and shoulders are fully extended. Repeat.

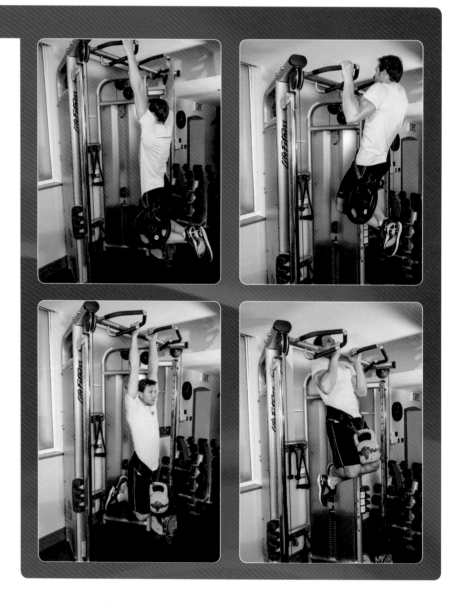

Weighted dips

Progression of dip

▶ Place weight on dip belt around waist or place dumbbell between lower legs. Climb onto dip bar, arms straight with shoulders above hands. Keep hips and knees bent and relaxed. Lower body by bending arms. When slight stretch is felt in chest or shoulders, push body up until arms are straight. Repeat.

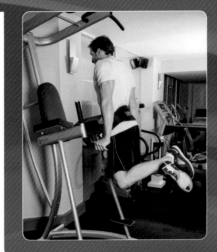
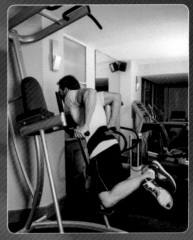

Weighted sit-up

Progression of sit-up

▶ Lie supine on the floor with a weight extended above the head on straight arms. Exhale and suck belly button inwards, while simultaneously flexing at the waist to raise upper torso from the floor. Keep lower back on floor and raise torso up as high as possible. Return until back of shoulders contact floor. Repeat.

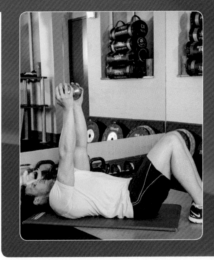
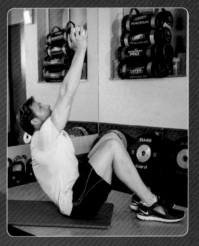

Wide grip upright row

▶ Grasp a bar with shoulder-width or slightly wider overhand grip. Pull bar up to front of upper chest with elbows leading. Allow wrists to flex as bar rises. Lower and repeat.

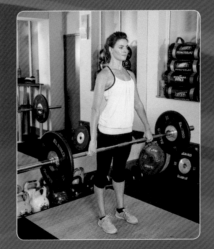
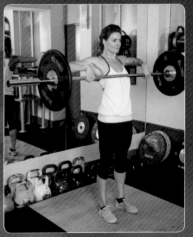

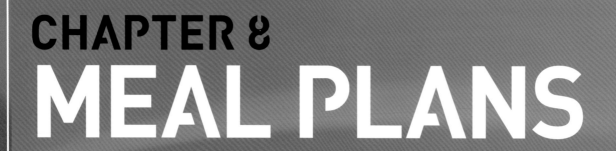

CHAPTER 8
MEAL PLANS

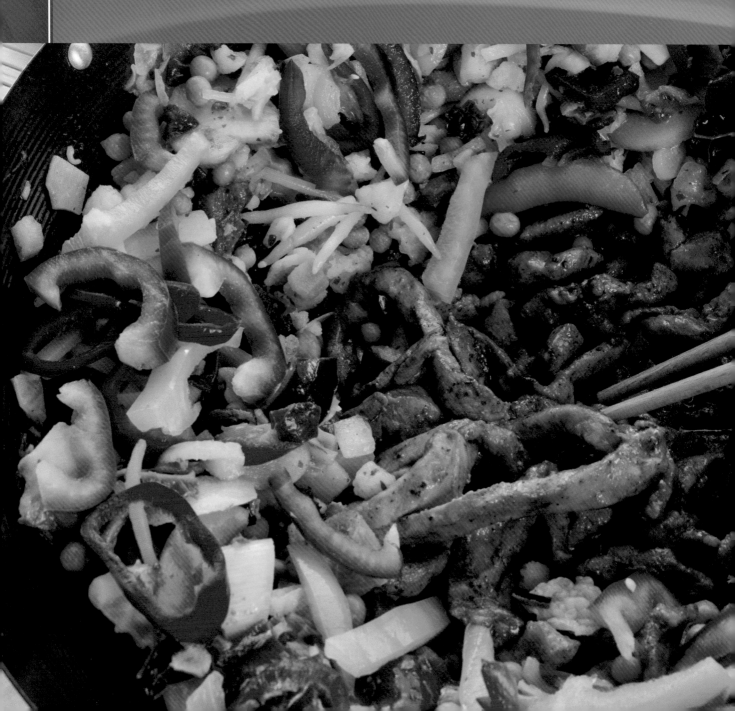

The following are just examples. They're meant to show you the timings and rough order of the various days' meals you could use over your 12 weeks, and then perhaps beyond. The meals may seem quite simple, but this is only because I've found that if I make the meals too complex there's a lack of compliance, and people soon fall back to High Street sandwich shops, thinking an extra LISS session will balance things out. Not so.

If you're a bit of a culinary master chef, feel free to liven things up and spend more time preparing your food – especially if it's something that'll inspire you and de-stress you. Again, if food preparation's a stress and not something you enjoy, then just get the basics done. You never know, it may grow on you!

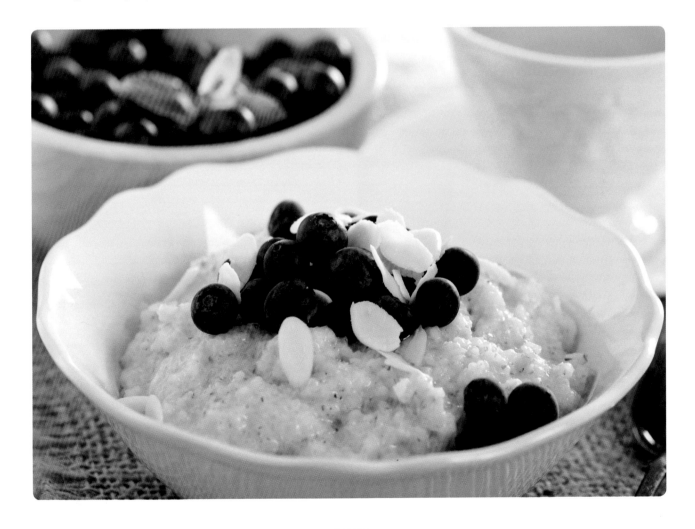

Example of a low (no) carb day

06:30 Pre-breakfast
Supplements:
1 x protein shake (20–40g whey).
1 x vitamin D.
1 x fish oil.
1 x CLA.
1 x vitamin C tablet.
1 x multivitamin.
(Morning LISS here, if in programme.)
Water.

07:00 Breakfast
Poached eggs and spinach.

10:00 Mid-morning snack
20–40g of whey.
Nuts (handful).
Coffee (not a latte). Black if possible. No sugar. If white, use a little whole milk or semi-skimmed.

13:00 Lunch
1 x mackerel fillet.
Half an avocado.
Baked kale seasoned with cayenne pepper.

16:00 Mid-afternoon snack
Chicken breast/turkey breast strips.
Broccoli/cauliflower florets.
Hummus.

20:00 Dinner
Chicken breast seasoned in chilli, ginger and olive oil.
Stir-fry bag with broccoli and cauliflower florets cooked in coconut oil.
Added chillies, if you're brave enough.
1 x fish oil.
1 x CLA.

22:00 Evening snack
FAGE Total Greek yoghurt and casein with blueberries.

Pre-bed
1 x ZMA or magnesium spray (eg BetterYou).

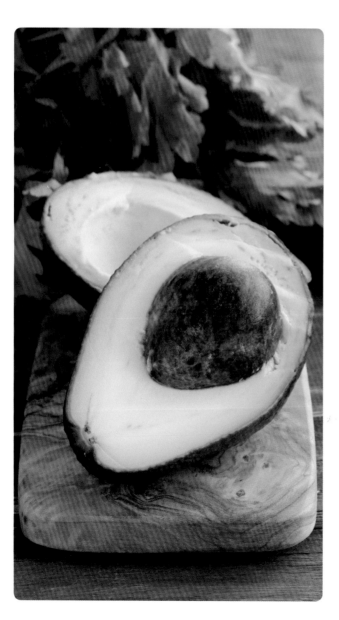

Note: FAGE Total Greek is given as it has the highest protein and lowest carbs of all I've seen on the market. Don't be tempted to buy supermarkets' own Greek yogurts, as they tend to have literally half the protein and double the carbs of Total. Whether you get the 0% or 100% comes down to how many calories you need personally. If they're quite low for what you've been used to, then 0%; if you're feeling like it's hard to get all your calories in, or you're an ectomorph trying to grow, then get the regular full fat version.

Example of a high carb day

06:30 Pre-breakfast

Supplements:
1 x protein shake (20–40g whey).
1 x vitamin D.
1 x fish oil.
1 x CLA.
1 x vitamin C tablet.
1 x multivitamin.
(Morning LISS here, if in programme.)
Water.

07:30 Breakfast

Porridge (made with water) with 30–40g whey, strawberries and raspberries.

10:00 Mid-morning snack

Sweet potato chips.
Turkey strips.
Broccoli and cauliflower florets.
Hummus or guacamole dip.

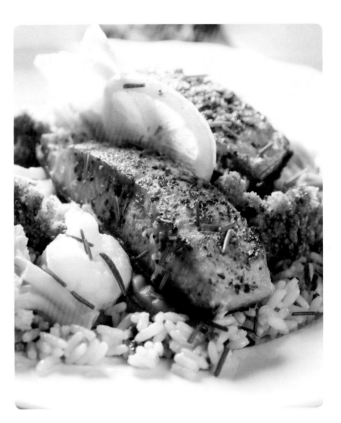

13:00 Lunch

Basmati rice (seasoned with coconut oil).
Salmon (seasoned with chilli flakes and ginger).
Spinach.

16:00 Mid-afternoon snack

Cottage cheese (low fat if calories need to be kept lower, but note carb content).
100% peanut butter.
Rice cakes.
Apple.

Pre-workout

20g whey.
5g creatine.
5g beta-alanine.

During workout

Water.

Post-workout

30g whey.
20g casein (or 10g casein and 10g soy).
5g creatine.
1 x banana.

20:00 Dinner

Sweet potato mash.
Turkey mince chilli (homemade sauce).
Kidney beans.
Peas.
Green beans.
1 x fish oil.
1 x CLA.

22:00 Evening snack

Porridge and casein with blueberries.

23:00 Pre-bed

1 x ZMA or magnesium spray (*eg* BetterYou).

Example of a medium carb day

06:30 Pre-breakfast

Supplements:
1 x protein shake (20–40g whey).
1 x vitamin D.
1 x fish oil.
1 x CLA.
1 x vitamin C tablet.
1 x multivitamin.
(Morning LISS here, if in programme.)
Water.

07:30 Breakfast

Poached or scrambled eggs.
Spinach.

10:00 Mid-morning snack

Chicken breast.
Celery sticks.
100% nut butter.

13:00 Lunch

Beef burgers (homemade if possible: from mince, with chillies and seasoning ground in).
Baked sweet potato.
Baked kale.
Apple.
1 x fish oil.
1 x CLA.

16:00 Mid-afternoon snack

Cottage cheese.
Rice cakes.
Avocado.

Pre-workout

20g whey.
5g creatine.
5g beta-alanine.

During workout

Water.

Post-workout

30g whey.
20g scoop casein (or 10g casein and 10g soy).
5g creatine.
1 x banana.

20:00 Dinner

Quinoa.
Tuna.
Broccoli.
Cauliflower.
Mixed beans/pulses.
Chillies.
1 x fish oil.
1 x CLA.

22:00 Evening snack

Porridge and casein with blueberries.

Pre-bed

1 x ZMA or magnesium spray (eg BetterYou).

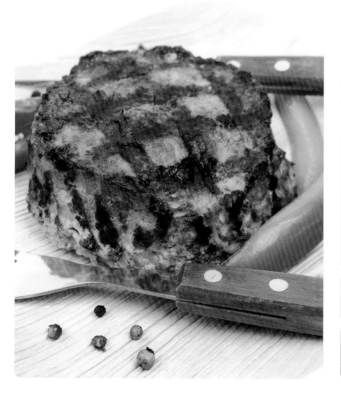

Food options and alternatives

The days outlined in the previous pages are just examples of the way you should try to structure your meals. By eating this way, it should help you keep things regular, and thus stop you reaching for the biscuits, sweets or chocolate, as you hopefully won't get any sugar crashes!

Equally, eating this way should ensure you have enough energy for your training, and won't break down any muscle tissue through lack of supplying the body with what it needs. Finally, by eating protein (around 20g) every three hours you should be able to keep your anabolic muscle synthesis switched on, thus helping you build more muscle, which in turn will help you burn more fat when you aren't even training. So that's a win-win.

Protein choice examples
- Chicken breast.
- Chicken thighs (with skin on, once or twice per week).
- Turkey breast.
- Turkey mince.
- Lean beef mince.
- Steak.
- Lean gammon.
- Lean ham.
- Lean pork.
- Tuna.
- Salmon.
- Mackerel.
- Sardines.
- Trout.
- Haddock.
- Cod.
- Pollock.
- Prawns.
- Crab.
- Eggs.

A palm-size portion of protein – *ie* one chicken breast, one tin of tuna etc – is around 20–25g of protein. This is a perfect benchmark for your 20g every three hours.

Dairy
- Total Greek yoghurt.
- Cottage cheese (high protein; fat content depends on your calorie needs – aim for as low carbs as possible, especially if having low fat version).
- Whole milk (better than skimmed or semi-skimmed, as more nutritious).

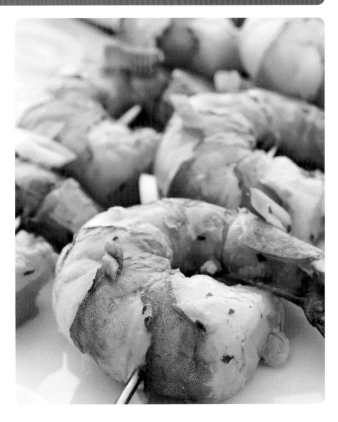

Protein supplements (See Chapter 5)
- Whey protein isolate (cold filtered concentrate if on a budget).
- Casein protein.

If lactose intolerant:
- Beef protein.
- Egg protein.

If vegetarian:
- Soya protein.
- Hemp protein.
- Pea protein.

Supplements – should-haves
- Multivitamin.
- Vitamin C.
- Vitamin D.
- Omega-3 fish oils.
- ZMA or magnesium spray.

Supplements – I advise you to have
- Creatine.

Supplements – nice to have
- Beta-alanine.
- CLA.

Carbohydrate choice examples

- Sweet potatoes.
- Porridge/oatmeal.
- Quinoa.
- Jasmine rice.
- Basmati rice.
- Rye crisp bread.
- Rice cakes.
- Wholemeal pitta bread.
- Popcorn (*not* salted/caramelised).

Obviously, there's a host of other carbohydrate sources out there, so just be sensible. Some are better than others, but the overriding factor is the amount of carbohydrate you ingest, which is why we worked out the amount of carbs you need per day. Keep to that amount and try to stick to the more 'naturally' occurring carbohydrate choices.

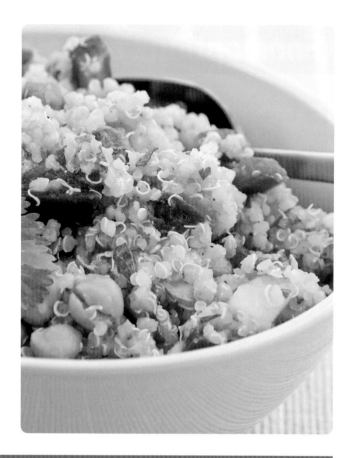

Vegetables choice examples

- Broccoli.
- Cauliflower.
- Bok choi.
- Spinach.
- Kale.
- Green beans.
- Asparagus.
- Peas.
- Brussels sprouts.
- Aubergine.
- Courgette.
- Squashes.
- Stir-fry bags.
- Mixed green salad.

Again, there's a myriad of choices available, and these are literally a handful of examples. If you have things you prefer, great, go with them. Just be aware of the overall carb value of them, and include it into your daily amounts. As stated earlier, MyFitnessPal for smartphones is a great tool to aid you with this.

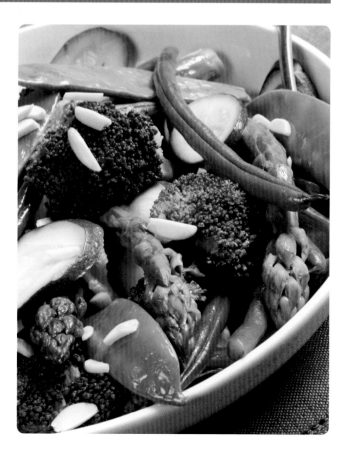

Fruit choice examples

(Don't go overboard on fruit – it's actually very sugary. Choose berries in preference to fruit if you have a sweet tooth or need a quick fix. Also, be aware that in terms of vitamins and minerals, vegetables are often a better and more nutritious choice.

- Blueberries.
- Strawberries.
- Raspberries.
- Blackberries.
- Cherries.
- Grapes.
- Apples.
- Bananas (post-workout only, as they release serotonin, which makes you feel sleepy).
- Peaches.
- Pears.
- Kiwi fruit.
- Pineapples.

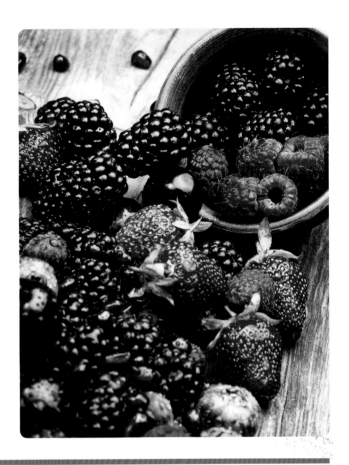

Once again, there are lots of different examples of fruits. Just ensure you stay within your carbohydrate allowance and don't use them as 'fast food' when you haven't prepared meals. The best bet with fruit is to top and tail your training sessions with it. My preference is an apple before and a banana after.

Fats choice examples

- Avocado.
- Fish oil capsules.
- Coconut oil.
- Olive oil.
- Fat from dairy.
- Nuts and 100% nut butters (no hydrogenated oils).
- Fish (oily fish like salmon, mackerel, trout, sardines especially).

As with the other macronutrients, there's a host of other foods in the fats group you could choose; just choose wisely. Remember,

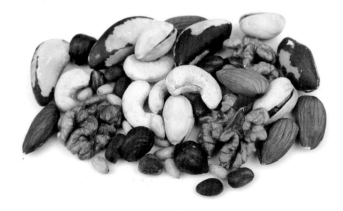

fats are 9kcal per gram so can soon add up. Also, try to avoid transfats as much as possible (found in commercially baked pastries, cookies, doughnuts, muffins, cakes, pizza dough and the like). Saturated fats from fatty cuts of beef, lamb and pork, chicken skin and whole-fat dairy products (milk/cream/cheese etc) get a bad rep. They're a good inclusion, but, like everything, should be used in moderation, and shouldn't be overdone.

There you have it. That's roughly the sort of foods you'll be eating over the next 12 weeks, and hopefully beyond. Well, there or thereabouts...

Again, the list is quite simple, and not overly restrictive or inclusive. I think you'll agree it's kind of middle of the road. As I said before, this is done so that it's not so restrictive that people don't conform, and not so inclusive that people go crazy. The point, yet again, is that everyone's different. For example, I can take more calories than Rachel McAdams, yet it's fair to say Chris Hemsworth (all 6ft 3in of him) can take more calories than me. We all need to be aware of our needs. Equally, I don't want 70–80% of the calories from fruit because I'm lazy and that's as close to pick-up-and-eat fast food as I can get. Put the time into preparing your food. Hit your protein needs; get some good fats into at least 25% of your daily calorie requirement and make up the rest of your calories with sensible carbohydrate choices like those I've listed.

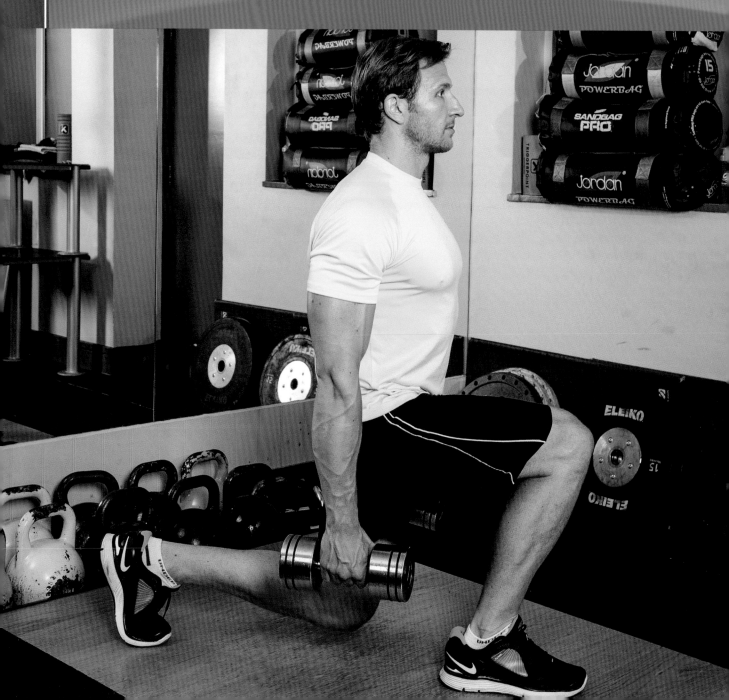

CHAPTER 9
TRAINING LOG

You might think that keeping a diary is just for teenage girls, people who hope to one day write an autobiography, or (in the fitness sense) professional bodybuilders. Well, you're wrong. If you really wish to succeed at changing your body, you're going to need to keep one too. I'd advise that it isn't just your training log, but also logs your food, supplements, sleep (or lack of), added stresses and, of course, your training.

If you log everything, it's far easier to see why (at the end of each month, or at the end of the entire process) you haven't achieved what you set out to achieve. And instead of throwing this book in the bin, it'll help you have another go, ensuring that you rectify the mistakes you made last time. Although I'm attempting to give you as much advice as I can, along with a training programme, guidelines for nutrition and all the other experience I can pack into a book, the simple fact is – as I've said before – that there's no one-size-fits-all solution. People are different. Full stop. This means their training is also different, and thus you may need to look back at your training diary, tweak the advice in this book so that it better suits your own needs, and repeat.

Logging

Whether you log in a notebook, or on your laptop, tablet, phone or whatever, just ensure that you do it. As we were told in the Marines, 'be as detailed as possible; you can never give enough detail'. When you look back retrospectively you won't remember things clearly, but if you write it all down at the time, giving as much detail as you can, it'll help you analyse your results and draw accurate conclusions.

Secondly, log everything as soon as you can. Some people actually carry a notebook, logsheet or their phone/tablet with them as they train. Personally I'm not a fan of this, as I find it a distraction. I also find it gets covered in sweat and I'm constantly worried about losing or breaking it. Therefore I log everything as I eat my post-workout meal. Again, it doesn't matter how, just ensure you do.

A picture paints...

In the Marines we were told that 'a picture paints a thousand words, so draw a diagram' – or in this case, take a picture. Weekly progress pictures taken from the front, back and sides will help you no end – I guarantee you won't see the changes

otherwise, as you see yourself every day, whereas comparing pictures taken six weeks apart will speak volumes. Ensure you take your weekly picture at the same time, in the same place, in the same light and wearing as close to nothing as you dare. If you travel a lot because of work, then fair enough, just do the best you can in the locations you're in; but otherwise wherever possible same place, same time, each week.

Weight

Although I don't advise it for everyone (especially women), weighing yourself can also be handy once a week when you take your photo, and this should be added to your diary. Again, ensure you take it at the same time and use the same scales where possible. I often find women get hung up about their weight as

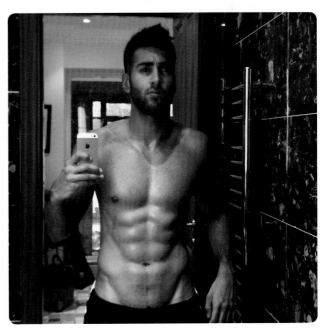

they undertake a body transformation, as they 'gain' weight. It doesn't matter that they've lost body fat and look (in the pictures taken) a thousand times better, all they moan about is weighing X kilos. But it's irrelevant what you weigh. Do you look better? Do you like what you see compared to the picture you took on day one? Yes? Then it's going well, right? Good, so forget about your weight unless you're planning on entering a fighting competition or becoming a jockey.

Measurements

Measurements can also be taken – around the belly button, thighs, upper arms, chest, neck and backside. Just use a normal tape measure around these areas. Either get someone to help you (the same person each time) or do it yourself. Note these

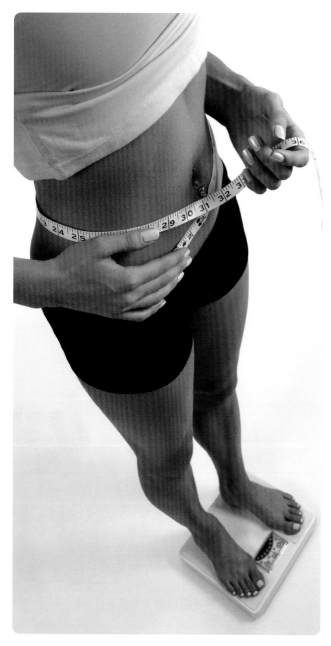

Avoiding plateaus

If everything stays the same, you stay the same. You have to continually challenge the body to ensure it keeps adapting. Logging everything you do allows you to force adaptations and avoid plateaus by never giving your body exactly the same session. Variation is key.

down each week in your diary when you have your photos taken: same time each week, if possible. The changes will then be documented for you to see, even if you don't feel you can see them yourself.

The importance of logging

Your goal of changing your figure or physique is of upmost importance during your 12-week training process. However, what happens when the results don't come quite as planned? Well, as I said previously, you simply tinker with the nutritional/training plan and attempt it again. The problem arises if you don't know *why* or *where* things went wrong. That's why you need to track and log everything in a training diary. Not only does this allow comparisons week to week, in terms of weights lifted, reps performed and so on, to allow you to gauge over training; it also allows you to track your progress.

You know already from reading this book that to ensure your body keeps transforming, compositionally speaking (body fat down, muscle percentage up), you also have to consistently challenge it: progress and ensure intensity. The problem comes if you can't remember what you did the last time you did this training day, or this exercise, or lifted this weight. What people do then is guess. This inevitably leads to using the same weights for the same reps – *ie* no progression, no intensity, and thus a less than perfect session. Again, that's where your training log comes in.

This book lays out your exercise selection(s), the number of reps and sets you should aim for, the tempo you should use to ensure adequate time under tension, and, of course, the amount of rest you should aim to take. Obviously your weight selection is down to you, but we need to ensure you're challenging yourself. As you know, if everything else is kept the same you need to increase the weight – hence looking back at your training log and making the necessary changes next time. It may be that another variable is changed: the rest times are decreased, tempo made more challenging etc, in which case the weights will stay the same. Same answer, though: look back at the training log to see what you did previously.

If you continually challenge your muscles by increasing the weight, reducing the rest, increasing the reps, adding more sets or introducing a more difficult tempo, you'll continue to force adaptations in the muscles while burning excess body fat. So log your training and ensure you're doing what's needed.

Example training log sheet

Exercise	Target reps	Target sets	Weight	Tempo	Rest	Actual reps	Notes
Monday							
1 Deadlift	10	3	30kg	4010	90sec		
2 Back squats	10	3	40kg	4010	90sec		
3 Overhead press	10	3	20kg	4010	90sec		
4 Bench press	10	3	35kg	4010	90sec		
5 Lat pull-downs	10	3	40kg	4010	90sec		
6 Push press	10	3	25kg	4010	90sec		
Tuesday							
Rest or Tabata sprints on treadmill/rower	20sec	8	NA	20sec/ 10sec	120sec		
Wednesday							
1 Deadlift	10	3	30kg	4010	90sec		
2 Back squats	10	3	40kg	4010	90sec		
3 Overhead press	10	3	20kg	4010	90sec		
4 Bench press	10	3	35kg	4010	90sec		
5 Lat pull-downs	10	3	40kg	4010	90sec		
6 Push press	10	3	25kg	4010	90sec		
Thursday							
Rest or Tabata sprints on treadmill/rower	20sec	8	NA	20sec/ 10sec	120sec		
Friday							
1 Deadlift	10	3	30kg	4010	90sec		
2 Back squats	10	3	40kg	4010	90sec		
3 Overhead press	10	3	20kg	4010	90sec		
4 Bench press	10	3	35kg	4010	90sec		
5 Lat pull-downs	10	3	40kg	4010	90sec		
6 Push press	10	3	25kg	4010	90sec		
Saturday or Sunday (not both)							
Rest or Tabata sprints on treadmill/rower	20sec	8	NA	20sec/ 10sec	120sec		

Exercise	Target reps	Target sets	Weight	Tempo	Rest	Actual reps	Notes
Monday							
Tuesday							
Wednesday							
Thursday							
Friday							
Saturday or Sunday (not both)							

Exercise	Target reps	Target sets	Weight	Tempo	Rest	Actual reps	Notes
Monday							
Tuesday							
Wednesday							
Thursday							
Friday							
Saturday or Sunday (not both)							

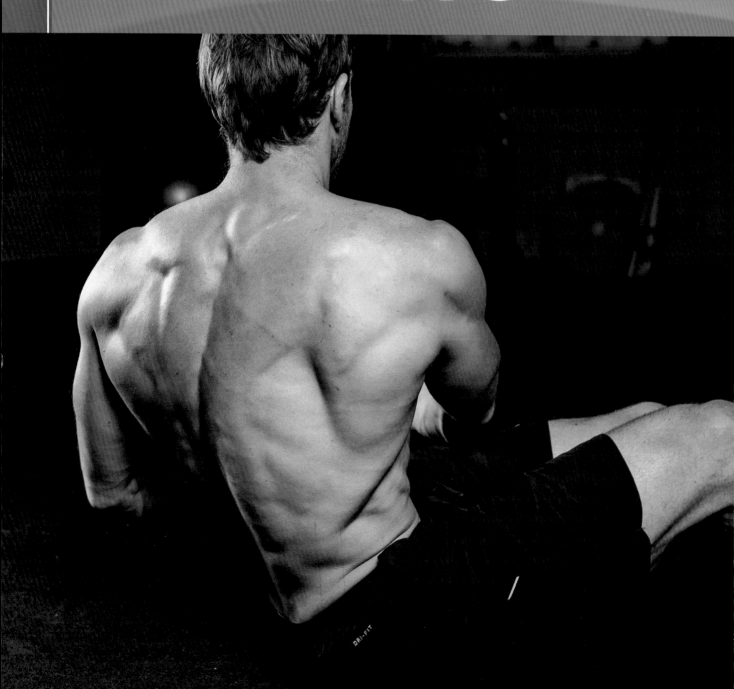

CHAPTER 10
CLOSING THOUGHTS

This final chapter comprises a few additional things that I thought might help you start or complete your journey, enhance it in some way, or maybe give you somewhere to go afterwards.

Transformation rules

1 Lower calories to lose

If, like most people who want to undertake a body transformation, you wish to burn fat and build muscle, we need to make sure you have a calorific deficit for the majority of the time. To do this, keep to the calories you've worked out for yourself using the formulas on page 49. Utilise carb cycling once you've reached a plateau from a calorie deficit diet alongside the training programme.

2 Raise calories to build

Building muscle is a calorie-consuming process. If you're not getting in enough calories for daily bodily processes and repair, then your body won't expend energy on muscle growth. When training to build, stick to the calories you worked out for yourself using the formulas on page 53. If you're a real 'hard gainer' and find this just isn't working, up this to increase your muscle mass by multiplying by a different activity factor.

As explained in the nutrition chapter, try to keep calories high on training days, but lower them on rest days, as your body is expending less energy. This will enable you to gain lean muscle rather than adding excess body fat.

3 Protein is primary

When changing your diet, the easiest trick is to increase your amount of protein. For a body transformation, whether your goal is to lose fat, gain muscle or, like most people, both, ensuring that you eat protein at every meal, including snacks, will help you no end.

Since muscle is made of protein, it should make perfect sense that to grow muscle you need to eat protein. Ample

protein. Research shows that when following a weight-training programme for any type of change, ingesting 2.5–3g of protein per kg is the most effective regime for building muscle.

Research also suggests that when a good portion of that extra protein comes from whey protein, its ability to ensure muscle protein synthesis remains switched on, as well as the ease of its use for people with busy lifestyles, ensures that better changes occur than without whey.

If in doubt, and if you change nothing else about your diet, try to ingest a portion of protein (20–30g) every three hours. Although, as described above, calories really do count overall in terms of amounts ingested, protein is more difficult for the body to convert and store as fat, so trying to gain a high percentage (about 40%) of calories from protein can be a great start.

Use whey and casein supplements if you're happy to, but ensure you eat a good amount of whole food protein sources, such as eggs, beef, chicken, fish and dairy. At the end of the day whole foods are better, despite the added benefits of supplements.

If you struggle, follow these simple guidelines:

- **Breakfast** – Eat eggs. Don't worry about the carbs, like toast, cereal or fruit. Don't just grab an apple if you're running late and call it breakfast. That's fast food. Know thyself! If you constantly run late, then have a few hard-boiled eggs ready in the fridge for whenever you find yourself short of time.
- **Meals** – If you find yourself too busy and are thinking about skipping your three-hour protein meal window, don't! Have a protein shake. Protein shakes aren't meal replacements (I'd rather you had whole food), but they're better than nothing. Just don't make it a habit!

- **Eating out** – Avoid pizza, pasta and rice dishes. They often contain little protein. Order steak, chicken or fish. Vegetables and a side salad accompany these well and are usually available on request.
- **Snacks** – Cakes, biscuits, chocolate or a piece of fruit aren't good snacks. You need to snack on protein: Greek yogurt, cottage cheese, chicken strips, beef jerky or nuts (not too many though, as they're quite calorific). As usual, if you're struggling have a protein shake, but don't let it become the norm.

If you can follow the above and nothing else, you'll lose more fat and build more muscle.

4 Carbohydrate – the Devil or the second coming?

Over recent years, people have realised that 'fat' isn't necessarily the evil food type we thought it was. We now understand that we require a decent amount of good fats to function and survive. With 'diets' like the 'Atkins diet' making headlines, thanks to it's following in Hollywood, carbohydrate has now become the outcast of the macronutrient world. However, it's not quite that simple.

Carbohydrates are important when trying to build muscle. If you're a hard gainer and starting skinny, then you NEED an energy surplus in order to grow muscle. Your body uses glycogen store levels (the form of carbs stored in muscles and the liver), to help determine your energy status and whether or not your body is stocked up and able to initiate protein synthesis. Furthermore, because every gram of carbs stored in the muscles needs water (around 2–3g per gram of carbs), glycogen pulls water into the muscles. The more glycogen, the more water; this stretches the muscle cell membranes, which in turn switches on processes that increase muscle protein synthesis and long-term muscle growth.

For anyone at the skinny hard gainer end, you need a good amount of carbohydrate, not only for the reasons above, but also in order to fuel your workouts. If you don't have enough carbohydrate and are training hard your body will have little available to fuel your workouts. Otherwise, with little body fat, your body is likely to break down muscle – the opposite of what you want.

In Chapter 4, for hard gainers (those requiring weight gain) we worked out your carb intake after protein and fats (30% of calories) had been worked out, as it constituted the remainder. However, as a rough guide, on training days aim for 4g of carbs per kg of bodyweight, while on rest days, to try to reduce fat gain, drop the carbs down to about 3.3g per kg.

For most people wanting to reduce body fat to achieve their transformation goals, carbs are a difficult best friend. You need them, but if you see them too much they'll lead you astray. As was discussed in Chapter 4, we have to limit carbs if body fat reduction is the goal, but we need to increase muscle mass, as it's our metabolic tissue. Hence we keep carbs low while your body

fat is still relatively high, then as it drops we carb cycle, so that we have high carb days (hard training days) to refuel our glycogen, help us feel normal and balance our hormone levels again.

We used the same method as described above, working out calories, protein and fat needs then making up carbs with what's left calorie-wise. However, as an idea, you should aim at 2.2g/kg per day on training days and as low as 1g/kg on rest days.

5 Fat to get lean

As I said above, fat is not the evil food source we once thought it was. Around 30 years ago there was a war on fat; dieticians recommended a very low-fat diet because a gram of protein or carbs has about 4 calories, but a gram of fat has about 8–9 calories. This means fat has twice the calories of protein or carbs. In addition it was assumed that fat makes you fat, and also leads to cholesterol and other health diseases. But in fact we need fat, even saturated fat, to maximise testosterone. Monounsaturated fat is equally critical in maintaining testosterone levels, as well as enhancing overall health. As already discussed, essential fats like omega-3s are crucial for muscle growth and joint recovery and help to lower body fat. So aim for 25-30% of calories from fat – about a third of that saturated fat, another third monounsaturated fat, and the final third polyunsaturated fat, with emphasis on the omega-3 polyunsaturated fats. Transfats are the man-made monsters of the macronutrient world and are the only fats that you should actively avoid. They're often found in baked goods, pastries, cakes etc. Avoid them wherever possible.

If you dislike oily fish or don't eat enough (once a day, or at least four times per week) then supplementing with 2–3g of fish oil two or three times per day can help.

6 Eat regular meals

Eating regularly is something that many people feel is counterintuitive, especially if they're trying to reduce weight/body fat. If you're skinny and want to get bigger, then it makes sense. As we've discussed, we need your body to create metabolic muscle tissue. We also want it to 'give up' the excess fat tissue, and eating regularly helps to do this, and especially to build muscle.

If you think of how babies and infants eat, they eat little and often, their whole purpose in life being to grow. Research has shown that 20g of protein ingested every two to three hours is the most beneficial way to add muscle, and, combined with a good training programme and calorific deficit, will therefore aid fat loss.

7 Breakfast

Breakfast comes from the term 'break the fast', because we don't eat during the 6–8 hours of night, which means that being asleep doubles the amount of time we usually go without eating protein (2–3 hours). The problem is that going that long without a meal can cause the body to break down muscle for fuel (brain

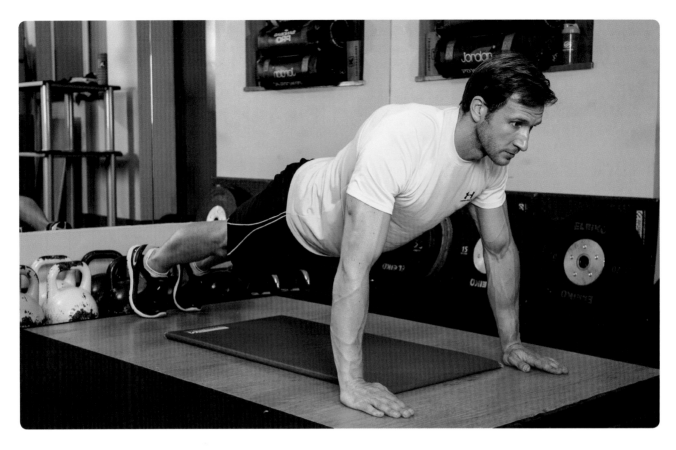

fuel and body repair while we sleep), which is the last thing you want when you're trying to build muscle to help you lower body fat.

The brain and central nervous system run on glucose (carbs). When you sleep, the majority of that glucose is supplied by the liver, which stocks up on stored carbs in the form of glycogen. When the glycogen levels of the liver reach a certain low point during the night, the liver signals the body to break down more muscle protein to convert the amino acids into glucose. You're asleep, so there's not much you can do (other than eating casein before going to bed). However, eating breakfast first thing will stop your body breaking down muscle to supply the brain, hence eating protein first thing is imperative. Having a whey protein shake will deliver amino acids quickly and stop muscle breakdown, which is why it's something I do almost every day.

If you're a 'protein shake first thing' person, then around 30–60 minutes after you should have a second breakfast of slower-digesting whole foods like eggs.

8 Eating to sleep

To minimise muscular breakdown when sleeping, it's a good idea to eat a slow-digesting protein before bed. In days gone by bodybuilders would set an alarm halfway through the night to get up and eat, but this isn't necessary. A good night's sleep is far better for growth and recovery, not to mention some of the hormonal changes that occur when the body isn't having to digest or process food.

As discussed in the supplements chapter, casein protein provides a steady supply of amino acids for around seven hours, which is perfect for overnight. Casein is slow-digesting because it forms micelles in the digestive tract, which are structured a bit like onions, with each layer of protein needing to be 'peeled off' and digested. This means a slow and steady stream of aminos is provided that stops the body from using amino acids from muscle breakdown to fuel the brain.

Besides casein supplements, Greek yogurt, cottage cheese or normal cheese (such as Cheddar cheese) could all be used in the same way. Research also suggests that some berries or fruit that refill your liver glycogen levels could also help casein-derived protein go even further, so having a handful of these – or, like I do, adding blueberries and casein to a bowl of porridge – should do the trick.

9 Eat your greens

When it comes to a body transformation, vegetables are arguably one of the most important things to eat. Not only will they help satiate you when you're cutting carbs or on low carb days, but they're also full of beneficial micronutrients (vitamins and minerals) and phytochemicals. These micronutrients help to promote better overall health, and help the body produce testosterone, growth hormone and nitric oxide (NO) to better promote muscle growth and thus fat loss. Furthermore, some top nutritionists believe that the acidity levels our foods produce when we eat them can also play a vital role in our overall health.

As eating high protein, and especially oats (one of the highest acidity ratings), raises acidity, it's important we level these off with alkaline foods: vegetables like kale and spinach are perfect for this.

10 Positivity

Keeping a positive mindset and avoiding negative thoughts, whether your own or projected by others, is imperative. If you want to achieve your goals, in life or in fitness, then a positive outlook has to be at the top of your list. You'll always have bad days, setbacks, failures and things that don't go to plan, and some people will let these stop them, get them down or make them quit. Successful people are those who react differently to failures, and this is often key to how successful they are. Remember the four elements of the Commando Spirit of the Royal Marines? – a sense of humour in the face of adversity is one of them. It may be difficult, but when things don't go your way try laughing, try to see the funny side. Try to imagine yourself looking back in a year's time when it doesn't matter any more. However you do it, remain positive as much as you can, and whatever you do don't listen to negative people who tell you it can't be done. Show them they're wrong.

> **If I can make you smile, I can make you happy. If I can make you frown, I can make you sad. Emotion, in this sense, goes outside-in.**
>
> Malcolm Gladwell

11 Worry about you

When you're in the gym, the only person you should be concerned about (unless someone starts having a heart attack) is you. Ignore the exercises other people are doing, what weights they're lifting, how bad they look, how good they look. Ignore the pretty girl or guy training across from you. Get on with your session, time your rests, lift your weights, get in and get out. Reap the benefits. Have a chat in the foyer, changing rooms, car park etc if you must, but in the gym *train*. People will respect you for it, none more than yourself.

12 Variation is key

People always want to know what the 'best exercise for abs is', or 'what the best exercise for upper pecs is'. As Dr Jim Stoppani says; 'The best exercise is the one you are NOT doing'; or as I say (repeatedly, because it's so important), 'Variation is key.' This goes for exercise selection as well as rep ranges and rest times. People worry about what 'the best rep range is for muscle growth'. The best rep range is the one that sees you fail when you perform a

good-quality exercise, with good form and using a good tempo. This will vary depending on the weight you use and rest time you give yourself. Variation itself has been shown by research to be more effective for muscle growth, strength gains and fat loss than any one specific rep range.

Although this book has a programme with varying exercises and reps ranges, if you wish to employ it with other exercises or types of training, simply decrease the rep range as you increase the weight every week over a four-week period: week one use 12–15 reps, in week two use 9–11 reps, in week three use 6–8 reps and in week four use 3–5 reps. You can then repeat that cycle with new exercises for the next four weeks. Simple periodisation.

13 Use intervals

There's a place for both LISS (light intensity steady state) runs and HIIT (high intensity interval training) runs. But if you're going to do nothing other than increase protein, follow a resistance programme and do *some* cardiovascular training, then choose intervals. Research shows that high-intensity interval training outperforms steady state for fat loss, performance, and cardiovascular health. (As I've said though, it does take a greater toll on the body, which is where LISS can be beneficial.)

A simple interval session can be created from any exercise, not just the normal swim, bike, run, row. Skipping, kettlebell swings, power cleans, box jumps, burpees can all be used. Tabata is a good option, but actually any 2:1 ratio of exercise to rest is great: 30-second intervals of high-intensity exercise alternating with 15-second intervals of rest, or one-minute intervals of exercise with 30-second intervals of rest, for instance.

14 Be active

Human beings used to be far more active than they are today. Before cars, TVs, office jobs etc we led far more active lifestyles. As kids, we were more active too, with PE and games being part of our lifestyles. But as adults most of us spend our days sitting at a desk. Research shows that this literally shuts off genes involved in fat burning, which results in your body slowing down its fat-burning. Therefore, be active. Go for a walk, play some sport, walk to work instead of driving, just don't be sedentary: don't get stuck in the rut of lying in bed, sitting in a car, sitting at a desk, sitting at lunch, sitting at a desk, sitting in a car, sitting in front of the TV, going to bed. Get some activity in every day. If you undertake this training programme fully, you'll be active. If you fall off the wagon, then keep being active every day until you can recommence.

15 Take a multivitamin

Before considering any other supplement, think about a multivit. Intense training leads to losing many critical vitamins and minerals (B, C, chromium, selenium, zinc, magnesium and copper) in sweat and urine. The amount of each you use also increases for energy production during training, and in recovery and protein synthesis post-training. Deficiencies in vitamins and minerals can decrease performance, fat loss and muscle growth, so take a multivit that has 100% daily value of most of the vitamins and minerals.

16 Treat meal

We know nutrition is 70% of the battle, so eating healthily is a must. You need protein, sensible carbs, vegetables and healthy fats to make you feel better, look better, perform better and live longer. But as we've said, being rigid 100% of the time will affect your glycogen storage, moods and hormones and therefore other factors. Equally, you only live once – you may want to look good, but you also want to enjoy life. Have a treat meal once every few weeks or each week depending on your body fat percentage. If you allow yourself to have the things that make you happy that one meal a week, or perhaps go out with friends once a week on a Friday, that will make this whole process more bearable. Also, it's a carrot to encourage you while you're working hard and eating sensibly all week. If you don't earn it, don't allow yourself to have it! A scheduled treat meal at the end of the week leads to better compliance. Not only is it something for you to earn and look forward to, it also gets the craving out of the system so that you can be good again for another week. A treat meal will cause no damage as long as you stick to your diet the rest of the time!

17 Partner

Most people find that when they train with a partner they train better and accomplish more. Whether it's down to healthy competition, or just the fact that a solo human will unconsciously choose a slightly easier path, partners motivate each other to do well. Strangely, it seems that productivity and effort when training with a partner increases, whether the partner or trainer actively gives encouragement or not – meaning you don't need a training partner who shouts in your ears to make you lift more! Simply being there will make you work harder (unless, obviously, they aren't really into achieving and are just trying to persuade you to hit the pub).

You and your partner need the same goals. The beauty of this is that the level of achievement is therefore far greater than can usually be attained when working individually. That word 'intensity' that I've repeated so often in this book can be injected by training with a partner. Put it this way, even Marine recruits who are highly motivated need others; so do Olympic athletes in training. Everyone has a low point or a bad day, and this is when their teammates, coaches, partners etc really earn their money or show their love and support. Working with a partner, you'll motivate, encourage and inspire each other to achieve more than you could alone.

Having said that, if you don't have a partner, don't worry. There are lots of forums and social networks where you'll find all the interaction you need, while still doing your sessions alone.

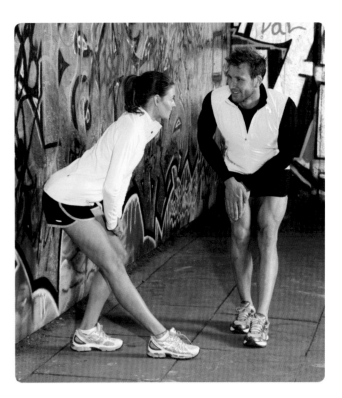

18 Intensity

It's that word again. I really can't emphasise enough how important intensity is. If your sessions are easy, they won't trigger any change. If they're easy, it's because they lack intensity. Try to push yourself each time. Imagine your transformation is being made into a documentary and the BBC cameras are on you. You'd do everything properly (technique, tempo), you'd choose the heaviest weights you could use and you'd still do things properly. You'd push for extra reps on every set. Simply put, you'd want to be the best version of you that you could be, for all to see. Well, that's what you have to do in each session. Remember, 'That'll do, will never do.'

19 Post-workout window

You know by now that, in general, high-sugar foods aren't great for achieving a six-pack. However, consuming sugar is actually good for you, and won't lead to fat gain straight after exercise, as during exercise you burn up glycogen. Glycogen is the body's storage form of carbs, stored in the muscles and the liver. These stores are depleted by exercise, and research shows that the best way to replenish these stores is by eating high-glycaemic sugars straight after training. Fruit is a good option, bananas are my personal favourite. However, if you have sweet cravings, you could eat sweets like 'Skittles' at this point, to stop you doing it at another point! The sugars would be good for muscle recovery and won't cause you to gain fat. Compliance-wise, having fruit or sweets after workouts can help you stick to the regime the rest of the time – just don't kick the ass out of it! A handful of Skittles, one piece of fruit or around 50g of dextrose/malodextrin is enough.

20 Where to go next

There are so many training programmes out there after completing this that it's hard to know what to do next. First, take a rest. Take a full week off to recover and let your body repair, recoup and adjust. Following this you could repeat the programme once again. From start to finish. If not, the following could be of use:

1 To gain strength

The '5 x 5' programme was designed to increase strength and break plateaus. Anyone with at least some training background would probably derive some kind of success from it.

Monday
Squats: 5 x 5.
Bench press: 5 x 5.
Bent over row: 5 x 5.
Accessory exercises: weighted sit-ups and a triceps exercise (note that these aren't compound exercises and are done to simply round out the programme. You don't need to follow the same 5 x 5 protocol as with the exercises stated above, and should do 2–3 sets of 5–8 reps).

Wednesday
Front squats: 5 x 5.
Military press: 5 x 5.
Deadlifts: 5 x 5.
Pull-ups: 5 x 5.
Accessory exercises: 2–3 sets of 5–8 reps of a biceps and abdominal exercise.

Friday
Squats: 5 x 5 (same weight as Monday).
Bench press: 5 x 5.
Bent over row: 5 x 5.
Accessory exercises: 2–3 sets of 5–8 reps of a triceps and abdominal exercise.

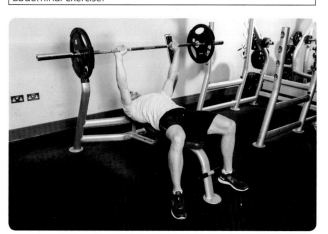

2 To gain size and strength

GVT programme 10 sets x 10 reps, one minute rest 4010 tempo. Splits.
- Day 1: Chest and back.
- Day 2: Legs and abs.
- Day 3: Off.
- Day 4: Arms and shoulders.
- Day 5: Off.

Day 1
Decline dumbbell press
10 sets, 10 reps, 4010 tempo, 90 seconds rest interval semi-supinated grip (palms facing each other).
Chin-ups
10 sets, 10 reps, 4010 tempo, 90 seconds rest interval (palms facing you).
Incline pec flyes
3 sets, 10–12 reps, 3020 tempo, 60 seconds rest interval.
Incline prone dumbbell row
3 sets, 10–12 reps, 3020 tempo, 60 seconds rest interval.

Day 2
Squats
10 sets, 10 reps, 4010 tempo, 90 seconds rest interval.
Leg curls
10 sets, 10 reps, 4010 tempo, 90 seconds rest interval.
Cable crunch
3 sets, 15–20 reps, 2020 tempo, 60 seconds rest interval.
Seated calf raise
3 sets, 15–20 reps, 2020 tempo, 60 seconds rest interval.

Day 3
Off.

Day 4
Bar dips
10 sets, 10 reps, 4010 tempo, 90 seconds rest interval.
Incline hammer curls
10 sets, 10 reps, 4010 tempo, 90 seconds rest interval.
Incline prone reverse flyes
3 sets, 10–12 reps, 20X0 tempo, 60 seconds rest interval.
Incline dumbbell lateral raise
3 sets, 10–12 reps, 20X0 tempo, 60 seconds rest interval.

Day 5
Off.

Repeat

3 To increase hypertrophy

Gironda's 8 x 8 – 8 sets of 8 reps on each exercise, only 30 seconds rest between, 3010 tempo.

Day 1	
Chest	Low cable crossover 8 x 8.
	Bench press 8 x 8.
	Incline dumbbell press 8 x 8.
	Dips 8 x 8.
Biceps	Hammer curls 8 x 8.
	Preacher curls 8 x 8.
	Incline dumbbell curls 8 x 8.
Forearms	Zottman curls 8 x 8.

Day 2	
Shoulders	Incline lateral raise seated 8 x 8.
	Wide-grip upright row 8 x 8.
	Bradford press 8 x 8.
	Incline prone reverse flyes 8 x 8.
Triceps	Kneeling triceps rope extensions 8 x 8.
	Skull crusher 8 x 8.
	Triceps kickbacks 8 x 8.

Day 3	
Back	Chin-ups 8 x 8.
	Incline prone dumbbell row 8 x 8.
	Low cable row 8 x 8.
	Medium-grip lat pull-down 8 x 8.
Abs	Sit-up 8 x 8.
	Cable crunch 8 x 8.
	Incline reverse crunch 8 x 8.

Day 4	
Quads	Front squats 8 x 8.
	Leg press 8 x 8.
	Sissy squats 8 x 8.
	Leg extensions 8 x 8.
Hamstrings	Lying leg curls 8 x 8.
	Leg curl 8 x 8.
Calves	Standing calf raise 8 x 20.
	Seated calf raise 8 x 20.

A final word

I hope this book has changed your life. The people I've transformed never go back to who they were before – partly because they prefer who they are now, partly because I like to educate and they realise how much healthier they are now, and also because getting to the end hurts, and the thought of throwing it all away is far worse! So, well done for reading this far, keep up the fitness life and be the best you can be. Be sensible, stick to the basics, try your best every day and if you suffer a setback, pick yourself up, take note of how it happened, and try again. No one gets anywhere without failure.

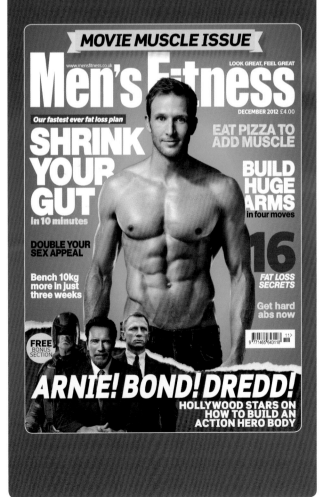

Glossary

Atrophy – A decrease in muscle size.

BCAAs – Branch chain amino acids.

Bodyweight – Exercise performed only with the body.

Burpee – An exercise which you start from a standing position before dropping into a squat with your hands placed on the ground; you then kick your feet back while keeping your arms extended, bring your feet back to the squat position and jump upright.

CLA – Conjugated linoleic acid.

Complex set – A series of back-to-back exercises with minimal or no rest.

Compound – An exercise that involves two or more joint movements.

CV – Cardiovascular.

DHA – Docosahexaenoic acid.

DOMS – Delayed onset muscle soreness.

Dropsets – Performing a set to failure with a chosen weight, then lowering the weight 20–30% and working to failure with that weight, then lowering the weight another 20–30% and performing to failure again.

EPA – Eicosapentaenoic acid.

GVT – German volume training.

HIIT – High intensity interval training.

Hypertrophy – An increase in muscle size.

Intervals, interval training or HIIT (high intensity interval training) – A form of cardiovascular training that requires the trainee to perform a series of high intensity repetitions interspersed with low intensity/rest periods. For best results, the high intensity intervals should be as close to maximum effort as possible. Forms of interval training vary from short bursts of 20 seconds' work and 10 seconds' rest (commonly known as Tabata training) to longer intervals of 1–2 minutes. The exercise itself can be cycling, running, rowing or swimming, or even static exercises such as skipping, kettlebell swings or the dreaded burpee, for example.

Isolation – An exercise that involves just one discernible joint movement.

LISS – Low intensity steady state.

Loading phase – A period of time needed to 'load up' on a supplement (*eg* creatine) so that the body is flooded with it before returning to a maintenance dose.

mTOR – Mammalian target of rapamycin.

RDA – Recommended dietary allowance.

Reps – Repetitions.

REST – Recovery equals successful training.

Rest/pause – A method of training beyond failure with a given weight: lift the weight to failure point, then rest for 1–15 seconds before lifting the same weight to failure again. This is often performed twice after initial failure.

Tabata training – Interval training composed of short bursts of 20 seconds' work and 10 seconds' rest.

Tempo – The speed at which the weight is lifted and lowered.

TUT – Time under tension.

Volume – Total amount of work performed in a training session.

Index

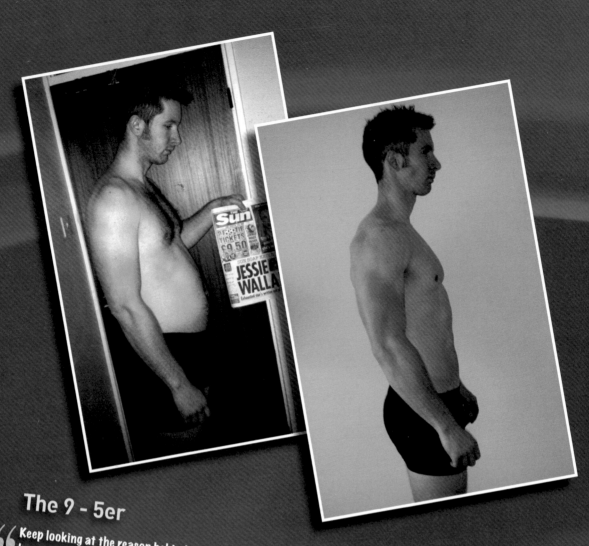

The 9 - 5er

" Keep looking at the reason behind the transformation to keep up the motivational levels.

For me I had two things that kept me going which are probably very different to why most people would do this. First being the future and wanting to be healthy for my son. Secondly, having a training partner and not wanting to let him down.

There was also a competitive element between us which I think helped both of us stick to things religiously. "

The Medical Student

" Give up the drink, gets rid of the unwanted calories and doesn't mess with your hormone balance. Also, prevents you eating crap that night or even the next day!

Check out your local gym first to make sure it has all the kit you need, especially the free weight section. Ask around and look on muscle/bodybuilding forums.

Have a few quick meals in your repertoire which you can quickly make if in a rush or on the go. Invest in some good Tupperware and prepare meals the night before to take for lunch.

You're making lifestyle changes, not one-off changes for the 12/14 weeks. "